BASKETBALL SHORT STORIES FOR KIDS

Charlotte Gibbs

© Copyright 2023 - All rights reserved.

The content contained within this book may not be reproduced, duplicated or transmitted without direct written permission from the author or the publisher.

Under no circumstances will any blame or legal responsibility be held against the publisher, or author, for any damages, reparation, or monetary loss due to the information contained within this book, either directly or indirectly.

Legal Notice:

This book is copyright protected. It is only for personal use. You cannot amend, distribute, sell, use, quote or paraphrase any part, or the content within this book, without the consent of the author or publisher.

Disclaimer Notice:

Please note the information contained within this document is for educational and entertainment purposes only. All effort has been executed to present accurate, up to date, reliable, complete information. No warranties of any kind are declared or implied. Readers acknowledge that the author is not engaged in the rendering of legal, financial, medical or professional advice. The content within this book has been derived from various sources. Please consult a licensed professional before attempting any techniques outlined in this book.

By reading this document, the reader agrees that under no circumstances is the author responsible for any losses, direct or indirect, that are incurred as a result of the use of the information contained within this document, including, but not limited to, errors, omissions, or inaccuracies.

TABLE OF CONTENTS

Introduction
6

CHAPTER 1
The Mailman's Missed Delivery—A Lesson in Basketball Pressure
8

CHAPTER 2
Harlem Globetrotters—A Slam-Dunkin' Tale of Basketball Magic!
12

CHAPTER 3
The Unbelievable Underdog—Why Villanova's Victory Is a Lesson in Believing
17

CHAPTER 4
Barkley vs. Rocky—The Hilarious Hoops Feud!
24

CHAPTER 5
Vince Carter's "Honey Dip"—A Dunking Dream
29

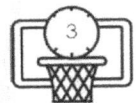

CHAPTER 6
Michael Jordan's Hoop Hijinks—The Curious Case of the Missing Jersey!
36

CHAPTER 7
The Unstoppable Allen Iverson
41

CHAPTER 8
Jerome Lane's Unstoppable Dunk—The Legend of "Send it in, Jerome!"
45

CHAPTER 9
The Legendary Coach—Pat Riley
50

CHAPTER 10
Sky High Glory—Liz Cambage's Epic Olympic Dunk
55

CHAPTER 11
The Superfan—Nav's Incredible Journey
62

CHAPTER 12
Bill Russell—The Giant Game Changer Who Dunked on Inequality
66

CHAPTER 13
Shooting for the Stars
71

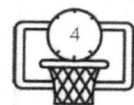

CHAPTER 14
The Unstoppable J-Mac—A Triumph of Dreams and Determination
76

CHAPTER 15
From Rookie to Champ—Magic's Mega Victory!
81

CHAPTER 16
The Hick from French Lick—Larry Bird's Left-Handed Game
88

CHAPTER 17
Linsanity Unleashed
93

CHAPTER 18
Mo Cheek's Most Memorable Assist
98

CHAPTER 19
Alonzo Mourning's Comeback—A Tale of Courage and Triumph in Basketball
102

CHAPTER 20
The Sneaky Shot Heard 'Round the Court
107

Conclusion
114

References
116

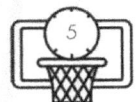

INTRODUCTION

Hey there, future hoop heroes and basketball enthusiasts!

Are you ready to lace up your sneakers, giggle through dribbles, and slam-dunk into a world of sporting legends and excitement? You are? Well, welcome to Hoop Heroes, where we'll embark on a court-side adventure like no other!

You might be wondering, "What's so special about basketball?" Well, guys, let me tell you a secret: basketball isn't just a sport; it's a playground for wacky surprises and jaw-dropping tales!

Picture this: a player shooting a wild air ball that somehow manages to tickle the referee's nose instead of landing in the hoop! And guess what? It's all true! Basketball is a game of laughter, fun, and lots of oopsies that make us giggle!

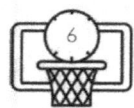

But hold up, it's not just about the funny mishaps. We've got some legendary slam-dunkers who soar through the air like superheroes. And trust me, you won't believe the incredible moments they've had on the court.

From a team of underdogs proving they're the real MVPs to a sneaky trophy thief who baffled everyone, these stories will leave you believing that in the world of sport, anything can happen.

And hey, it's not just about the game; it's about friendship, courage, and coming back stronger when the going gets tough. These ballers will teach you a thing or two about teamwork and sportsmanship.

So, grab your popcorn (or maybe some nachos), find a comfy spot, and get ready to dribble, dunk, and laugh out loud with the Hoop Heroes crew!

Are you pumped? I know I am! So, let's hit the court and dive into the most entertaining basketball journey ever.

Game on!

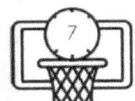

CHAPTER 1

THE MAILMAN'S MISSED DELIVERY—A LESSON IN BASKETBALL PRESSURE

In the world of basketball, there are players with awesome nicknames that make them even more legendary. You've got Michael "Air" Jordan, Earvin "Magic" Johnson, and Allen "The Answer" Iverson.

But let's talk about Karl "The Mailman" Malone. Since his college days, he's been famous for "always delivering" on the basketball court. He had an incredible career with the Utah Jazz, making it to fourteen All-Star Games and earning two MVP awards. "The Mailman" scored a jaw-dropping 36,928 points in his 19 seasons, putting him second on the all-time scoring list, right behind Kareem Abdul-Jabbar.

But one Sunday in June 1997, something unusual happened. Karl Malone faced a real lesson from Scottie Pippen during Game 1 of the NBA Finals against the Chicago Bulls.

With only 9.2 seconds left in the game and the score tied at 82, Malone had a chance to give the Utah Jazz the lead when he was fouled by Dennis Rodman. He headed to the free-throw line with everyone holding their breath, ready for some intense basketball action.

Scottie Pippen, who was known for his playful trash talk, decided to play a little mind game with "The Mailman." He whispered in Malone's ear, "The Mailman doesn't deliver on Sunday." And guess what? Pippen was right. The U.S Postal Service doesn't usually deliver mail on Sundays!

Karl Malone had already made three out of four free throws that night, but when he took his first shot, it didn't go in. With the pressure mounting, he tried to regroup before his second attempt. But unfortunately, lightning struck twice. His second shot had the same fate as the first—a clank! The Chicago crowd roared with excitement as the Bulls grabbed the rebound with 7.5 seconds left in the game. Too exciting!

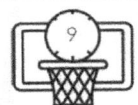

With the ball back in the hands of Michael Jordan, the pressure was on again. Jordan, the league's MVP from the previous year, took the final shot and made a 20-foot jumper over Bryon Russell at the buzzer. Chicago won the game 84-82.

In the end, even the greatest players can feel the heat when the game is on the line. It's a valuable lesson for all of us—sometimes, we face tough situations, and it's okay to feel nervous. What matters is how we handle the pressure and keep working hard to improve.

So, let's cheer for "The Mailman" Karl Malone, who always delivered, even on days when the pressure was sky-high. Even on Sundays! And let's remember that in basketball and in life, we can all learn from our challenges and come back stronger than ever.

So when things get tough, don't give up. Face challenges with a brave heart, and remember, they're like stepping stones that help you reach success. Think of "The Mailman" who never gives up delivering mail, because each time he tries, he gets closer to his goal. Keep trying, and you'll find the way to make your big dreams come true!

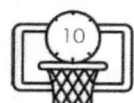

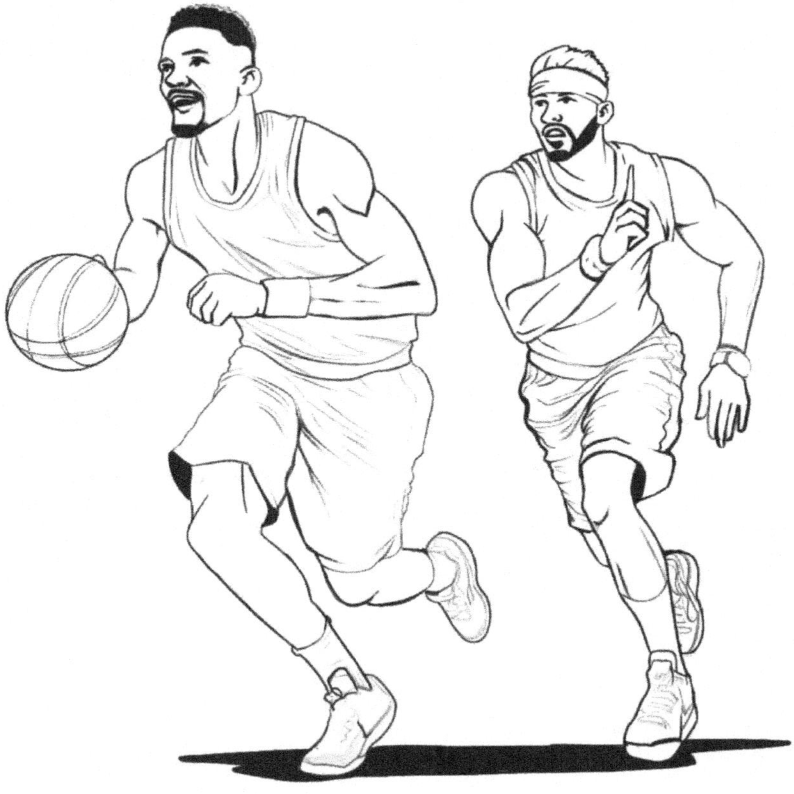

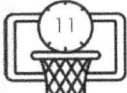

CHAPTER 2

HARLEM GLOBETROTTERS—A SLAM-DUNKIN' TALE OF BASKETBALL MAGIC!

Gather 'round, young ballers, for a side-splitting adventure with the Harlem Globetrotters and their uproarious journey through basketball history. Way back in the day, in 1927, these hoop-savvy wizards burst onto the scene, but let's rewind even further to the 1890s when basketball was just a baby born out of the YMCA. These guys were all about spreading kindness and making the world a better place through sports.

As basketball grew up, some stellar African American players hopped on the bandwagon, determined to slam-dunk racism while showing off their jaw-dropping talent. It was their way of saying, "Hey world, check out our balling skills!" Hold onto your giggles, because here's a funny fact—those Globetrotters weren't actually from Harlem! I

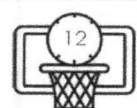

know, right?! The team was like a cool group of basketball superheroes from Chicago, but they called themselves "Harlem" and traveled around places like Illinois, Iowa, and Wisconsin, kind of like a group of buddies going on an adventure, showing everyone their cool moves.

Imagine this: a long time ago, there wasn't any NBA yet, and the Globetrotters were like the rockstars of basketball. They played games against all sorts of teams, on all kinds of courts—some were black, some were white, and some were all the colors! But in some places, things weren't very fair, and they had different audiences. But here's the cool part—the Globetrotters were like magic wizards when it comes to basketball. They did fancy moves that looked like spells, making the ball dance like magic! It was like watching two wizards have a cool spell battle, but with a basketball instead of wands! Move over Harry Potter!

Now, fast-forward to the late 1940s, when they took on the NBA champs, the Minneapolis Lakers. The Globetrotters whooped them in two games straight, and that might've nudged the NBA toward inclusivity. Can you believe it? And, even cooler, they shouted loud and clear: "Skills trump skin color!"

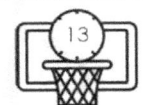

Now, here comes the funny part: back in the middle of the 1930s, the Globetrotters decided to be comedians too! They sure were a talented bunch. And they knew it! But how did they bring laughter into basketball? Well, imagine a super chilly game in Canada, where the air felt frostier than ice cream. The mood was serious, like a library during a quiet time. But then, like magic, they started doing crazy tricks and silly jokes with the basketball. And guess what? The crowd laughed so hard they almost fell over! This was something new! They turned into basketball jokesters, making people laugh and bringing divided communities together through a mutual love of sport and comedy! I mean, everyone loves to smile, right? These guys won the hearts of so many with their unique gifts of talent plus the ability to connect to their audience and connect others at the same time.

As the decades rolled on, the NBA was calling them, and some Globetrotters joined the big leagues. But did that stop the laughter? Nah! They kept up their jokes, spreading smiles all around, and throwing basketball parties worldwide. These jokers even welcomed amazing women players, like the enchanting Lynette Woodard in 1985. She spun her basketball spells with a grin that lit up the court.

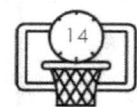

And so, the Harlem Globetrotters had their names written into basketball history, a mix of skill and fun. They taught us that b-ball isn't just about scoring; it's about spreading joy, high-fiving pals, and twirling the ball with a blinding smile. And that, my friends, is how the Harlem Globetrotters made a legacy that keeps surprising and impressing kids like you around the globe. So, shoot those hoops, dazzle with your dribbles, and sprinkle that basketball magic wherever you wander. Game on, and may the laughter never fade!

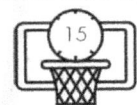

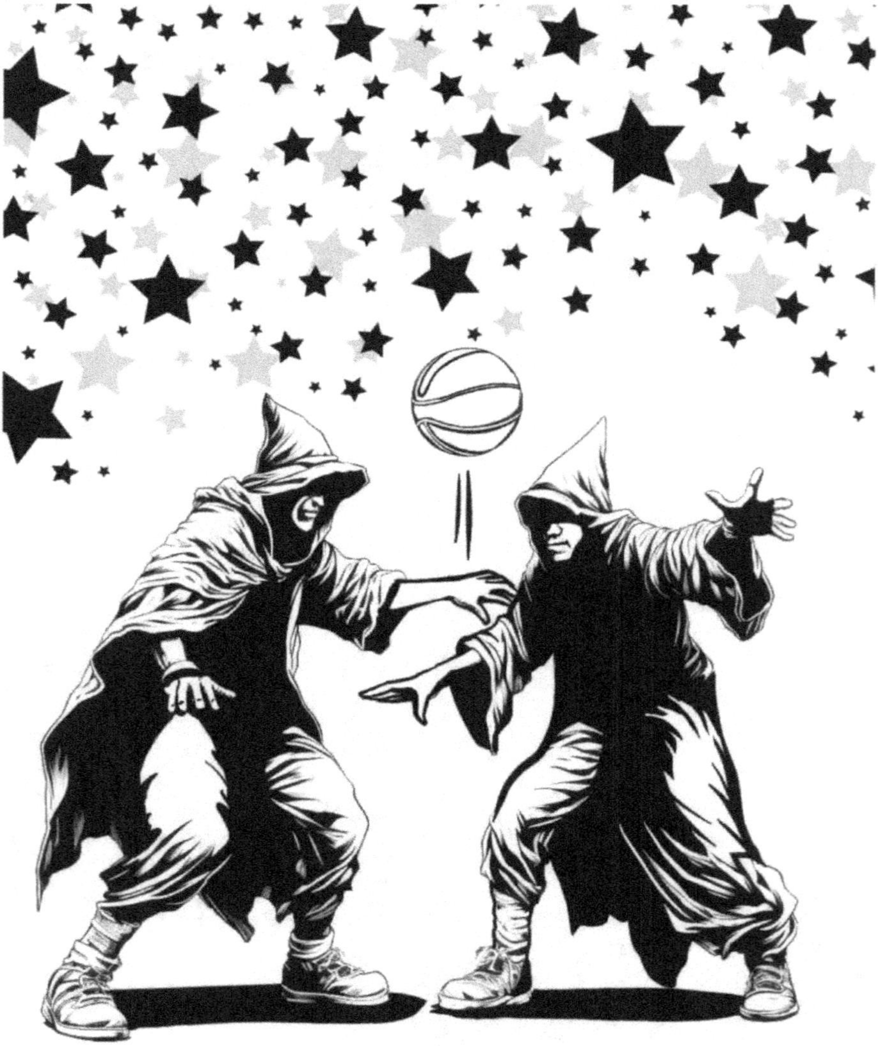

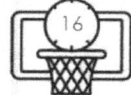

CHAPTER 3

THE UNBELIEVABLE UNDERDOG— WHY VILLANOVA'S VICTORY IS A LESSON IN BELIEVING

April 1st, 1985, was a magical night in college basketball history. The Villanova Wildcats took center stage in one of the most unforgettable basketball games in history. Their opponent was the mighty Georgetown team, led by the legendary Patrick Ewing. The Wildcats knew they were the underdogs, but they had a secret weapon—their non-stop belief in themselves.

The Wildcats, with their fan-favorite coach Rollie Massimino, had a plan for a perfect game. They knew it was their only chance against the powerful Georgetown Hoyas. Before the game, Coach Massimino told his players, "We'll need a perfect game to win, boys. Let's show them what we're made of!"

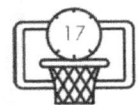

As the game began, the Wildcats played with heart and passion, matching the Hoyas point for point. Dwayne McClain, a senior forward, led the way with 17 points. The team's game plan was brilliant: they slowed down the pace, stopping Georgetown from getting on a scoring roll.

Throughout the game, the Wildcats shot the ball perfectly. They seemed to make every shot count, shooting an amazing 79 percent from the field. It was like watching a magical spell being cast upon the basketball, guiding it easily into the hoop.

But the magic didn't end there. The Wildcats also played a strong defense, challenging every move of the Hoyas. They even got Patrick Ewing, the towering center, into foul trouble, and stopping his flow.

With every pass and every shot, the Villanova crowd grew louder and more excited. The underdogs were showing the world that they could play with the best of them. Their secret weapon was their belief—they believed in themselves and in each other, and that made all the difference.

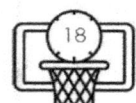

As the final seconds ticked away, the scoreboard read 66-64 in favor of Villanova. The crowd held their breath, watching a moment that would go down in basketball history. With just a few seconds left, Dwayne McClain tripped and grabbed the inbounds pass like it was a treasure. He shot his left fist skyward as the buzzer sounded, and the stadium started cheering with joy.

The Wildcats had done the impossible. They had beaten the mighty Georgetown Hoyas, a team that many thought were unbeatable. Coaches everywhere were inspired by Villanova's underdog story, using it as an example to motivate their teams. "Boys," they'd say, "let me tell you a story about a basketball game back in 1985."

The victory not only made Villanova basketball champions, but it also changed lives. For Toby Jensen, a sophomore on the team, it was a big turning point. He overcame his self-doubt during the tournament and made the most important shot in Villanova history. That shot also shot up his confidence and led him to doing well off the court as well. Years later, Toby started his own marketing company, Showtime Enterprises, using all the perseverance he learned during that championship season.

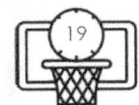

Xavier Pinckney, the spidery center, also found success after that magical night. His outstanding performance in the tournament made him the 10th pick in the NBA draft. After a long and successful professional career, he went back to Villanova as an assistant coach, passing on the magic of the game to a new bunch of players starting out.

The 1985 Villanova team became such close buddies that would last for the rest of their lives. To this day, they are still an unusually close group of players. Even after 30 years, they come together, sharing laughter and memories of their incredible journey.

The Wildcats' victory wasn't just about basketball. It was about believing in yourself, being proud of what is uniquely special about you, and never giving up, no matter how tough it gets or how unlikely you are to win. The game taught the world that with heart, determination, and a little sprinkle of magic, the underdogs can rise to greatness.

As you start on your own basketball journey, (or any journey at all) remember the magic of that night in 1985. Look at your strengths and be proud of them, believe in yourself, and never be scared to dream big. Whether you're

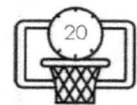

shooting hoops with friends or playing in a championship game, let the spirit of Villanova's win show you the way to your own dreams.

Basketball is more than just a game; it's a journey of growing stronger in all ways, of spending time with friends and helping each other, and of learning about yourself, what you're good at, what you need to improve on, and who you are – maybe you're a funny type, of a thinker, or maybe you love to make others smile. Be the underdog who shows that miracles can happen. Be the teammate who helps others either by doing things to help them out of just by making them laugh or smile or feel more confident and be the player who never gives up. And in every win and every loss, remember the importance of fair play, sportsmanship, and the magic of believing in your skills.

So shoot for the stars, young basketball players, and let the magic of the game light up the fire in you. Your journey has just begun, and who knows, one day, you might create your own legendary moment that inspires the world.

Never forget the power of determination and teamwork. It can be the biggest weapon ever! Just like the Villanova

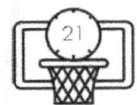

Wildcats, who faced incredible odds, you too can overcome challenges by believing in yourself and working together toward a common goal. To win, at whatever that may be. Celebrate the underdog spirit, for it is in those moments that you have the chance to shine the brightest. Celebrate every win, big or small, and remember that with perseverance and working together, you can do even what seems to be impossible. So, dream big, give it your all, and let your unshakable spirit lead you to triumph!

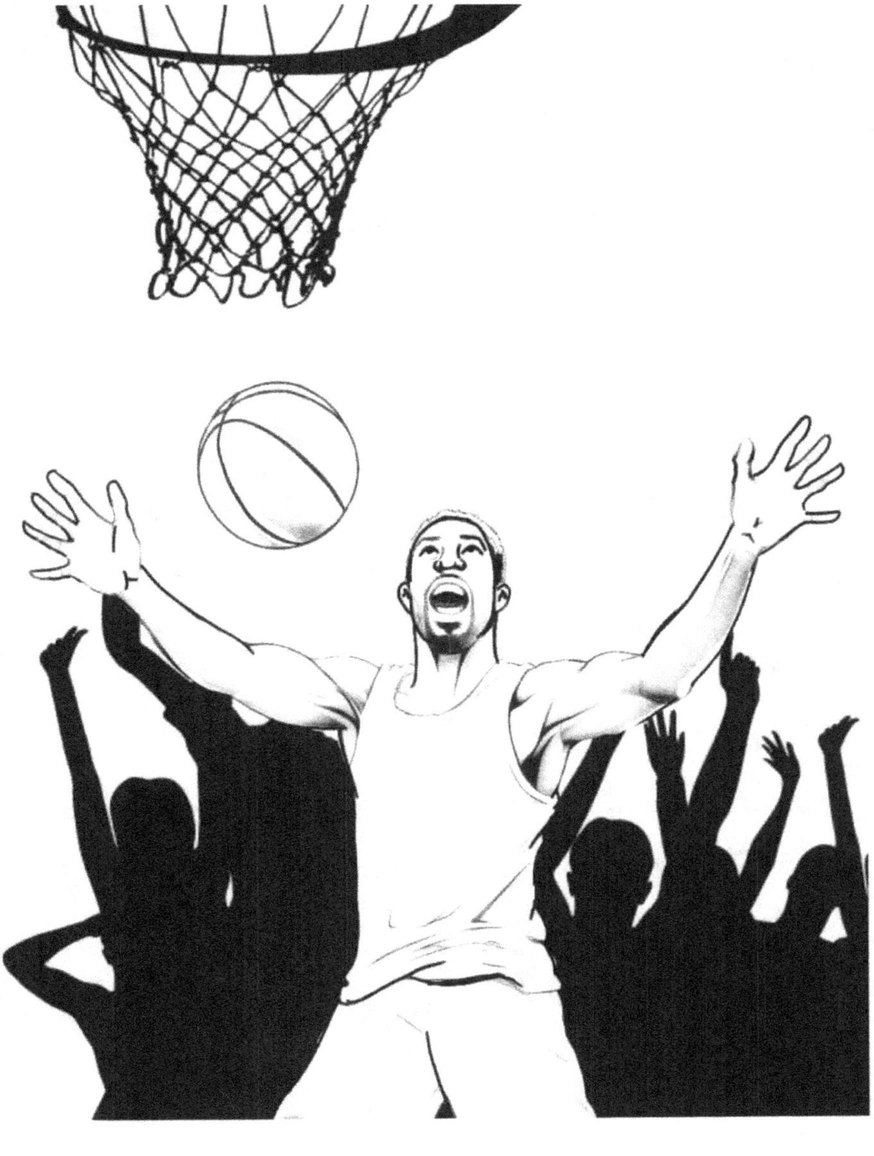

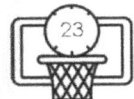

CHAPTER 4

BARKLEY VS. ROCKY—THE HILARIOUS HOOPS FEUD!

The lights went down in the arena as tales of epic battles between NBA legends were whispered into hushed ears. Then suddenly, a mischievous mascot burst onto the court, spreading chaos and mayhem that sent waves of roaring laughter through the stands.

Let's dive into the funny world of Charles Barkley and his epic battle with the Denver Nuggets' Rocky!

Back in the day, there was a famous basketball player by the name of Charles Barkley.

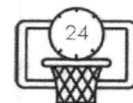

He was known for being super talented on the court and for being a bit of a hothead too! Yep, he had a temper. But guess what? The Denver Nuggets had a secret weapon—their mascot, Rocky! This cheeky little fella had a mischievous side and loved teasing Barkley.

Back when Barkley played for the Phoenix Suns, Rocky found so many ways to annoy him during games. It was like a funny dance of taunts and tricks! Fans couldn't stop giggling as Barkley's fierce glare was directed at the playful mascot, who was always one step ahead!

But wait, the tale doesn't end there! At one point, it seemed like Rocky wanted to make peace with Barkley. They exchanged jerseys as a sign of a new start. Oh, how sweet! But guess what? Rocky couldn't resist a sneaky move and gave Barkley a playful poke before darting away! Chuck was left chuckling, and the battle continued!

Now, kids, this isn't the first-time feuds like this have happened in the NBA. Devin Booker had his own funny beef with the Toronto Raptors' mascot in the 2020–21 season. But unlike Barkley and Rocky, Booker and the mascot patched things up quickly.

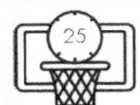

Charles Barkley, despite being the "Round Mound of Rebound" at 6'4, was an incredible basketball force! He outplayed players twice his size and earned a shiny MVP award. What a little legend! It's like he had some kind of superhero skills! Maybe he had a cape tucked into his jersey?!

Chuck's journey took him from the Philadelphia 76ers to the Phoenix Suns, where he became a superstar. He led the Suns to glory in many seasons but couldn't quite grab that championship ring. Nevertheless, he was a hero on and off the court.

Nowadays, Barkley is not just a basketball legend but also a much-loved hilarious broadcaster on TNT's "Inside the NBA." Picture him joining a wild and wacky panel, cracking jokes left and right! He's like the wizard of comedy and analysis of the game!

So, my little hoop enthusiasts, remember that even NBA legends like Barkley can have a silly side. Battles with mascots can be as fun as the game itself, warming hearts and bringing smiles to everyone! It's important to take our sports seriously, or anything seriously that we care about, and want to do well in, but we can remember too, that having fun, bringing smiles to others, and enjoying life is what it's all about. So, let's keep laughing, playing, and enjoying the magic of basketball adventures. May the laughter never stop on and off the court!

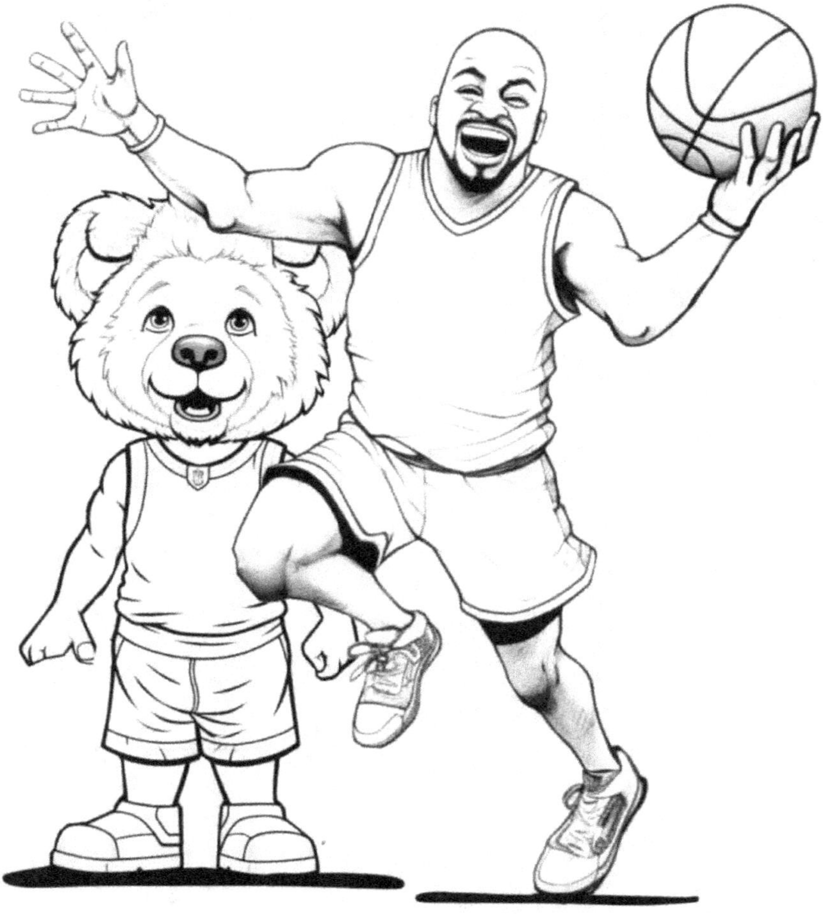

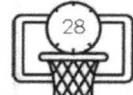

CHAPTER 5

VINCE CARTER'S "HONEY DIP"—A DUNKING DREAM

Vince Carter, who played for the Toronto Raptors, was known as "Half-Man, Half-Amazing." He had a reputation for jaw-dropping dunks that left everyone shocked at his skills. But there was one dunk that would go down in history as the "Honey Dip."

It all happened at the NBA All-Star Weekend in the year 2000. The Slam Dunk Contest had lost a bit of its shine in recent years, but Carter was about to change all that with his incredible performance. The crowd was buzzing with excitement as Vince stepped onto the court, ready to show off his aerial skills.

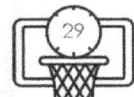

With a flick of the wrist, Vince started his magic with a ridiculous 360 windmill dunk. The crowd erupted into cheers, and everyone knew they were in for a treat. The energy in the arena was buzzing and the crowd was on the edge of their seats.

Next up, Carter displayed a slightly changed copy of J.R. Rider's famous "East Bay Funk Dunk." With some help from his teammate and cousin, Tracy McGrady, Vince took flight and soared through the air like a superhero.

But the most awesome moment came when Carter attempted the "Honey Dip." He dribbled toward the hoop with style and power, getting faster as he got closer. With a leap that did not seem possible for us flightless humans, Vince soared toward the rim like a majestic bird.

The audience held their breath as they watched history in the making. Carter's arm stretched out like a helicopter's rotor, and he hung in the air like a basketball wizard. He had done the impossible—he hung from the rim by his arm after the dunk, a feat never seen before in the NBA Slam Dunk Contest.

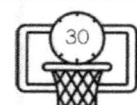

As he landed, the crowd erupted into a frenzy of cheers and clapping. Shaquille O'Neal, Steve Francis, and Jason Kidd stared in amazement. Kenny Smith called for a timeout, unable to process what he had just witnessed. Even Isiah Thomas couldn't contain his laughter at the brilliance of Carter's dunk.

The Slam Dunk Contest had come alive once again, and it was all thanks to Vince Carter and his "Honey Dip." With that dunk, he had changed the game forever.

Throughout his career, Carter was known for his SportsCenter-level dunks. His All-Star appearances and incredible athletic abilities had people comparing him to the legendary Michael Jordan. But on that magical night in 2000, Vince created a legacy of his own.

The Slam Dunk Contest was never the same after that. Carter's victory set the bar impossibly high, and no other dunk could match the skill of that evening. In following years, contestants tried all sorts of gimmicks and props to impress the judges, but nothing came close to the raw brilliance of Carter's dunk.

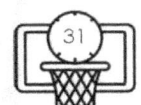

As time went on, the Slam Dunk Contest lost some of its shine once again. Many people said they should end it once and for all, as it struggled to live up to the unforgettable performance of Vince Carter. But in the hearts of basketball fans, that night would always be a special memory of what the Slam Dunk Contest used to be.

Vince Carter's crazy "Honey Dip" dunk reminds us that in life and in sports, there are moments that leave us breathless and amazed. Moments where we think, how did that happen?! Moments like these bring a spark to our daily lives. They remind us that wonderful and surprising things can be just around the corner and that can keep us going during hard or boring times. Just like Vince, who soared through the air with style and power, you too, can reach for the stars and never be afraid to push the boundaries of what you can achieve. Never think there are limits to what you can do. Look at your unique talents, be proud of them and use them to make a big impact on the world around you, and help inspire others, just like Vince did with his unforgettable dunk. Remember that greatness is not achieved overnight; it takes dedication, hard work, and a feeling of trying always to do your best, to be the best. So, dream big, set your sights high, and let nothing hold you back. And just like Vince's "Honey Dip" dunk left a legacy in basketball history, let your actions and

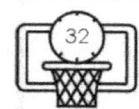

things you do well leave a positive mark on the lives of others. Believe in yourself, trust in all you can do, and keep striving for greatness, for the sky's the limit when you dare to dream and put your heart and soul into making those dreams come true.

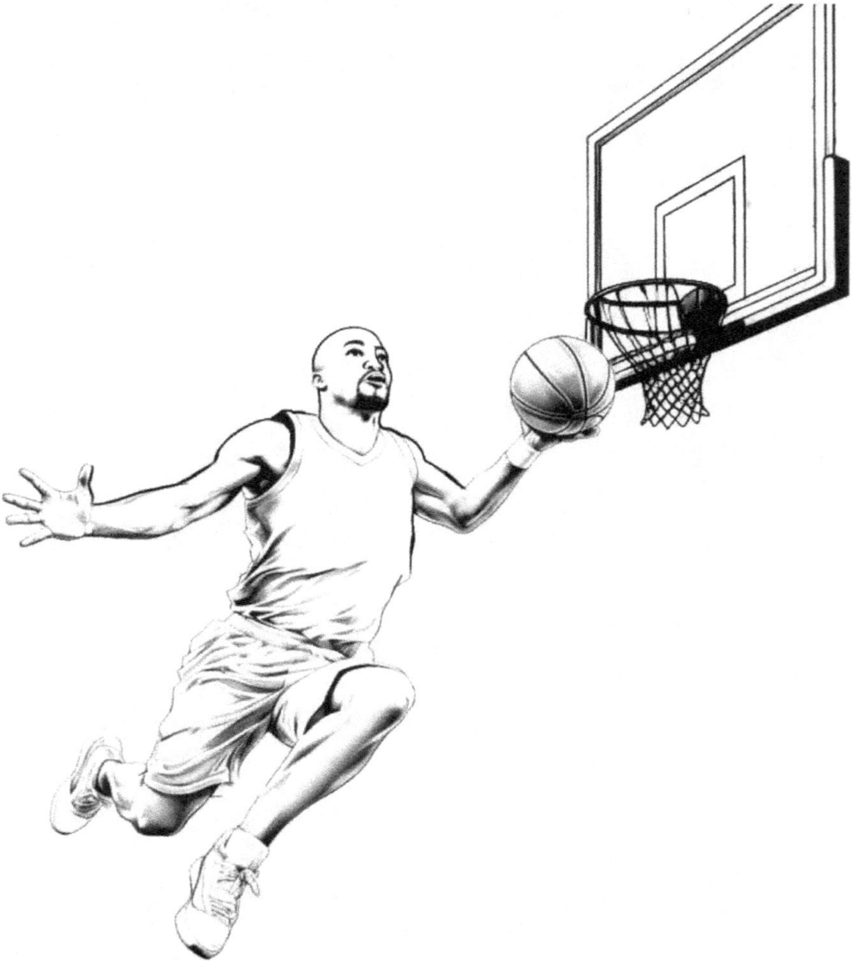

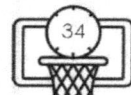

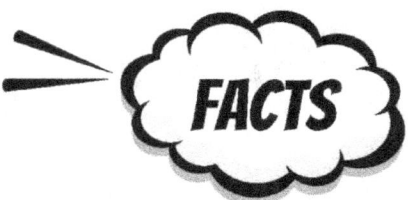

FACTS

1. Dr. James Naismith created basketball in 1891 to keep his students busy inside during the winter. They made use of a soccer ball and a peach basket.

2. The biggest player in NBA history is Gheorghe Mureşan, who is 7 feet, 7 inches tall.

3. The ban on dunking: In the early days of basketball, dunking was illegal because it was thought to be unfair.

4. WNBA Pioneers: The Women's National Basketball Association (WNBA) was started in 1996 to give women the chance to play professional basketball.

5. High-Scoring Games: The highest-scoring NBA game in history was in 1983 when the Detroit Pistons encountered the Denver Nuggets. The total score was 186-184, which was a shock!

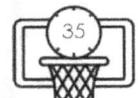

CHAPTER 6

MICHAEL JORDAN'S HOOP HIJINKS—THE CURIOUS CASE OF THE MISSING JERSEY!

Alright, gather 'round, my hoop-loving pals, for a mind-blowing tale from the NBA vault! It's all about the legendary Michael Jordan, but wait, this isn't your ordinary basketball story.

Picture this: it's the '90s, and Michael Jordan is already stacking up awards like rookie of the year, MVP, and defensive player of the year. But one fateful Valentine's Day, something mysterious happened. His super-famous number 23 jersey went missing from the locker room without a trace! Poof, gone!

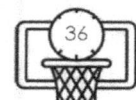

The Chicago Bulls were all set for a game against the Orlando Magic, but MJ's jersey was nowhere to be found.

The staff at the stadium searched the seats and aisles, madly running up and down stairways, looking between benches, and checking under the concessions stand. Yet somehow, the jersey was gone without a single sign of where it could be!

You might be wondering, what's the big deal? Doesn't he have spare jerseys? He's Michael Jordan! But you see, back in the day, teams traveled lightly to save money. They didn't carry much around. Those were the simple days! So, they brought only one uniform per player, and no backup jersey was available for the missing #23.

But fear not, the basketball universe had a surprise in store. The Bulls equipment staff found a spare jersey, but here's the kicker—it had no name, just the number 12! Who would have thought that the GOAT himself would wear a nameless jersey!

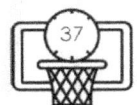

When Michael found out his jersey was stolen, he was crazy-mad! But guess what? The basketball wizard didn't let the annoyance or his bad mood or his bad luck get in the way of the game. He instead turned it into a show-stopping performance. He scored a whopping 49 points that night, taking a mind-boggling 43 shots; the second most shots he ever took in an NBA game! Now, that's impressive on its own, but when you think he pulled that off after a stressful time, it's something pretty awesome.

And guys, let me tell you, it was a sight to see! The arena was buzzing with excitement as the GOAT, wearing the mysterious number 12, dazzled the crowd with his magic moves!

Though the Bulls lost that game in overtime, the mystery of Jordan's missing jersey was never solved. It was like a real-life basketball mystery that had everyone scratching their heads. Someone, somewhere out there, has Michael Jordan's jersey! Maybe it will turn up one day... and if it does, it sure will have a story to tell.

So the next time you're watching a basketball game, and you see number 23 on the court, remember this tale

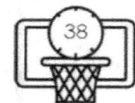

of the day it went missing, and Michael Jordan became the basketball wizard in the number 12 jersey! You can remember how he went on to play a massive, impressive game despite the drama right before it started. If you can leave your problems and stresses behind you and are able to focus on what's happening right now, whether it's an important game, a math test, or just a fun activity you've been planning but had some drama right before it, you can learn to leave it behind and still do well. Not only well, but you can really shine!

And who knows, maybe there's still a secret basketball detective out there, ready to crack the case of the missing #23 jersey! Until then, let's keep enjoying the magic of basketball and all the fascinating stories it brings.

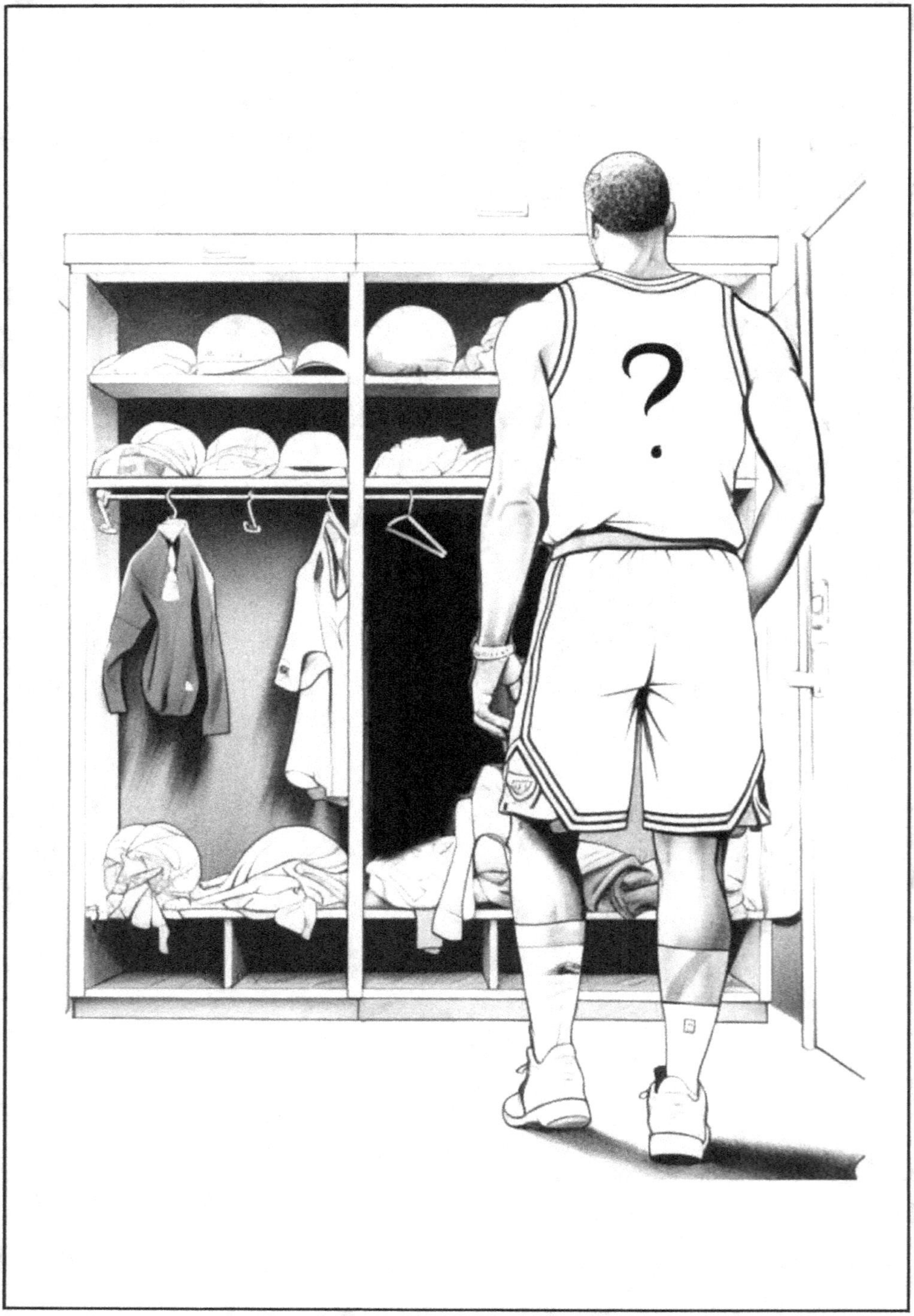

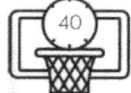

CHAPTER 7

THE UNSTOPPABLE ALLEN IVERSON

Get ready to meet a basketball superstar whose story is cooler than an ice cream truck on a summer day! Imagine a player named Allen Iverson, who rocked the court and had a journey full of twists, turns, and some serious high-flying fun.

Okay, so Allen grew up in a neighborhood where the sidewalks were tougher than a game of tag with super speedy cheetahs. But guess what? He fell in love with basketball faster than a shooting star zips across the sky. Even when he was just a tiny basketball sprout, he had moves that made everyone's jaws drop. His love of basketball was like a light that shone happiness on his tough, grey world. It kept him going!

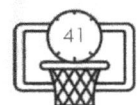

As he grew up, life threw some tricky curveballs at Allen. It was hard. But did he back down? Nope! He worked hard, practiced, and turned into a basketball star. When he played, it was like he had a secret stash of basketball magic up his sleeves. He even played for different teams, but his heart belonged to the Philadelphia 76ers—because he saw them as his basketball family.

Hold onto your popcorn, because here comes the funny part. When Allen was younger, he had a little event with a bowling alley that got him into a bit of a pickle. But guess what? He didn't let that stop him. He turned it around and used it as fuel to become even more awesome.

One day, his future knocked on his door, and Allen got a golden ticket to play at Georgetown University. He grabbed that opportunity faster than you can say "slam dunk," and he became the team's leader. His moves on the court were like secret codes that only he knew, and that's how he got the nickname "The Answer"; he always had the solution to any problem!

Then, ta-da! The big leagues arrived: the NBA. Allen was like a real-life superhero battling the bad guys on the court. He even went toe-to-toe with the legendary Michael Jordan, showing everyone that he was a basketball force to be reckoned with. He had what it took to be a star!

But Allen didn't just bring basketball skills to the table. His life story was like a lesson in never giving up, even when life gets as tricky as a maze made of spaghetti. Is that even a thing? Well, it is now! Anyway, he showed us that no matter where you start, you can reach the stars if you believe you can. He showed us that while all around you might feel dark, if you love something, and are good at it, grab it and make it a shining light for yourself.

So, all you awesome kids out there, remember Allen Iverson's story when things get wobbly. Whether you're facing math homework or climbing your own basketball mountain, know that with passion, effort, and a sprinkle of basketball spirit, you can achieve anything. Allen Iverson isn't just a basketball legend; he's your buddy that wants to show that you've got the power to shine, no matter what!

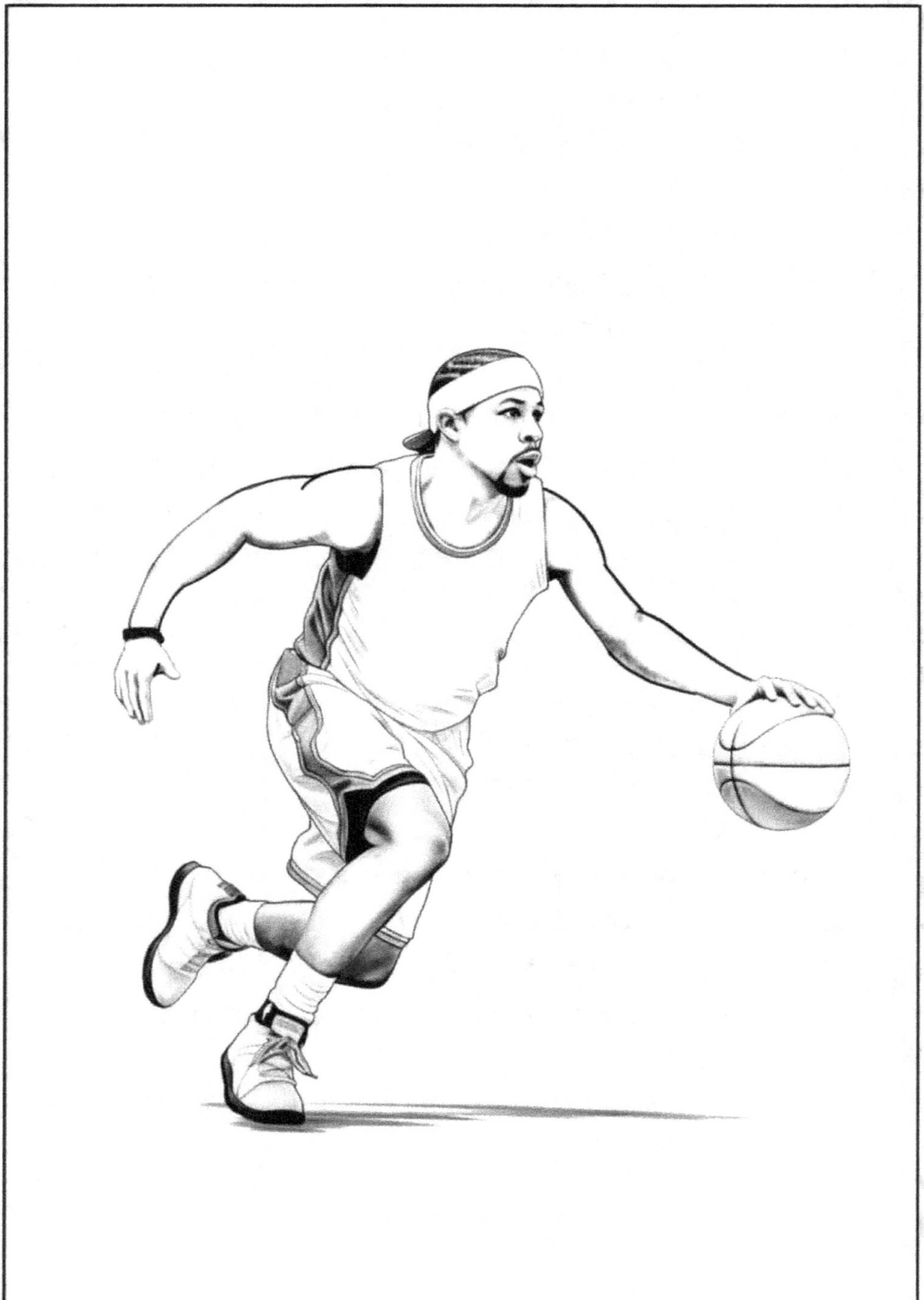

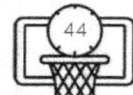

CHAPTER 8

JEROME LANE'S UNSTOPPABLE DUNK—THE LEGEND OF "SEND IT IN, JEROME!"

Oh boy, do I have a story that's sure to blow your basketball-loving minds! It's all about a jaw-dropping dunk that rocked the court and sent the basketball world into a frenzy!

Have you ever heard of the player named Jerome Lane? He was strong, fast, and had a secret talent for grabbing rebounds like a basketball ninja! But what he did next was something nobody could have expected.

It was a chilly January night in 1988, and Jerome was playing for the Pitt Panthers against Providence. The game was intense, and Jerome was pumped up to show off his basketball skills. He got the ball from his teammate, Sean Miller, and with lightning speed, he zoomed towards the hoop.

With one mighty leap, Jerome soared through the air like a basketball superhero and SMASHED the backboard with a monster dunk! Can you imagine the sound? It was like a light bulb going POP! The crowd gasped in shock. Did they really see what they thought they saw?!

But here's the best part - ESPN's Bill Raftery, the legendary announcer, was so amazed that he shouted, "Send it in, Jerome!" Those four words became famous instantly, like a special phrase that captured an unforgettable moment. A phrase that would lift anyone up if they heard it!

Everyone was in shock, including Jerome himself! But you know what's crazy? He couldn't do it again, no matter how hard he tried. It was like the basketball stars matched up perfectly for that epic dunk, and it could never be done again. Perhaps it was just too special!

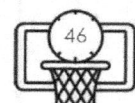

You know what? The game was actually paused for 32 minutes while crews searched for a new backboard. Imagine the players brushing glass shards from their hair! It was like a basketball adventure gone wild! Epic is the word we'd use to describe it these days.

In the end, the game was back on track with an old hoop that didn't even have a shot clock. The organizers must have been freaking out, but hey, the fans loved it! And Raftery had a surprise guest, a former NBA coach Don Nelson, to keep everyone entertained during the delay.

From that day on, "Send it in, Jerome!" became a basketball legend. It was like a magical phrase that ESPN and Raftery used to pump up college basketball fans all around the world! You know, what? You can use the phrase to pump yourself up any time you need. Try it! And if you love it, why not write it on a post-it and stick it somewhere you'll see it every day?

Even 25 years later, people still talk about that incredible dunk. Jerome and Raftery both became famous for that moment, and the basketball world cherishes the memory.

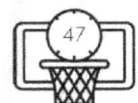

It's like a piece of basketball history that will never fade away.

So, my hoop-loving friends, the next time you're on the court and feel the basketball magic in the air, remember the tale of Jerome Lane and his unforgettable dunk. And who knows, maybe one day you'll create your own basketball magic (or even off the court magic) and leave the world in shock, too!

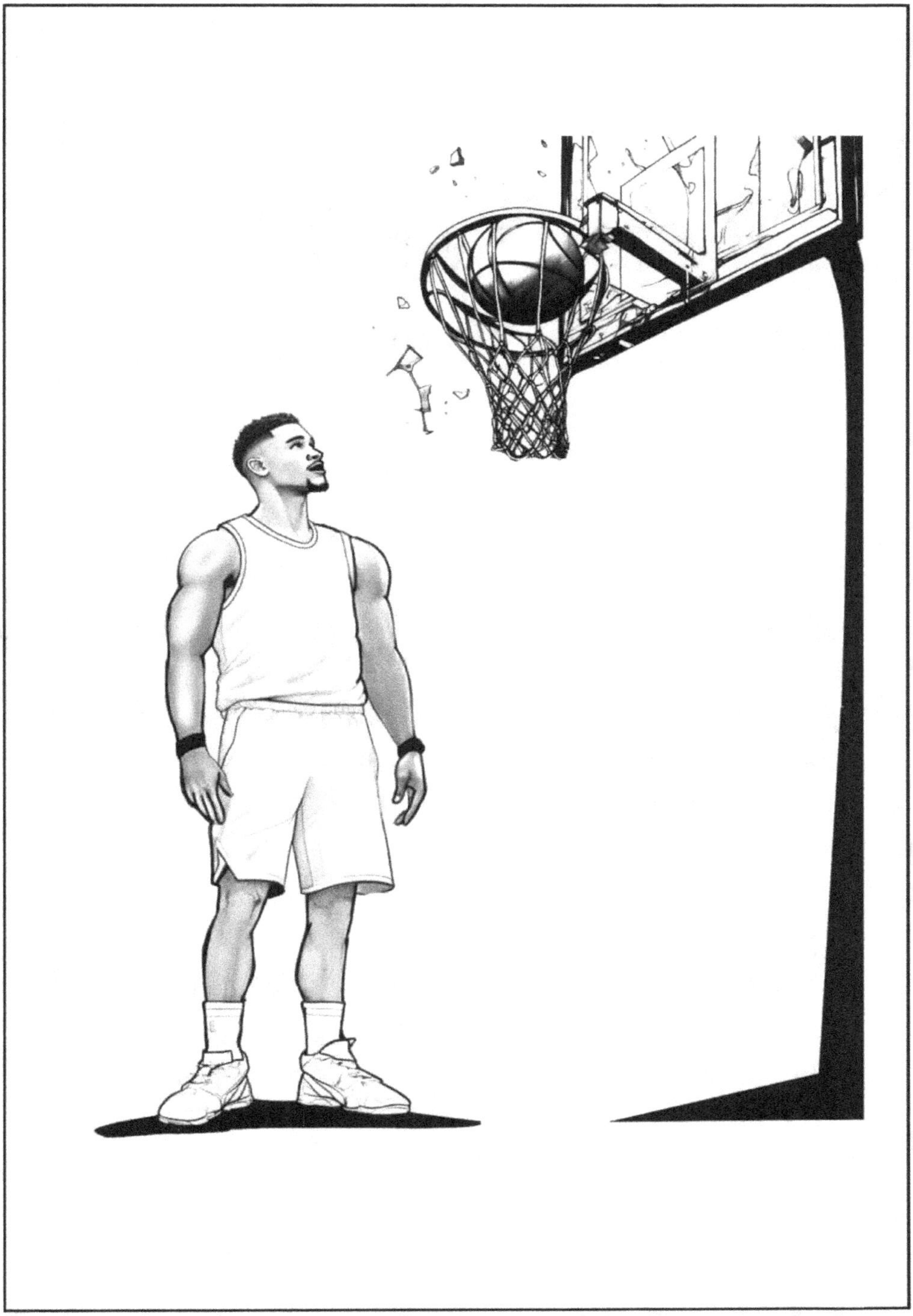

CHAPTER 9

THE LEGENDARY COACH—PAT RILEY

Step right into the world of basketball, where a wizard of strategy and a master of winning ruled the courts. Imagine someone who had the playbook of victory tattooed on their brain and could turn a losing game into a winning symphony. That someone was none other than Pat Riley, the ultimate maestro of the game!

Now, Pat wasn't just a basketball coach; he was a game changer, a name that meant one thing: winning. He had a taste of victory as a player, dazzling the world with his moves, and being part of the Lakers' record-breaking spree. But hold your popcorn because the real magic was yet to happen.

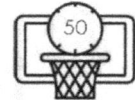

When he put on his coaching hat, things got wild! He had this thing called Showtime, and it was like watching a fast-paced circus of basketball tricks. Passes that defied physics, plays that made defenders dizzy—it was like basketball ballet. And guess what? The Lakers scored not one, not two, but four NBA championships under his winning spell.

But Pat's journey was a roller coaster. He switched teams and strategies like a kid flipping through a comic book. With the Knicks, he brought a tough, gritty style to the game, making them contenders even against the Bulls' basketball bulls.

Then, Miami called his name, and he knew the secret sauce: a dominant center. So, he brought in Shaquille O'Neal, a giant who was like a mountain with sneakers. And just like that, the Heat sizzled, winning the NBA title like they were collecting souvenirs.

But wait, the story wasn't over! Even as a team president, Pat kept weaving his basketball magic. He convinced LeBron James to join the Heat, and bam! Two more championships, like double scoops of winning ice cream. Very yummy indeed!

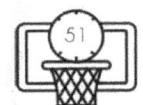

Now, hold onto your sneakers, because Pat Riley's career was like a movie where the hero never gets tired. He was a shapeshifter, who was able to change with the times. His secret? Hard work and discipline, kind of like superhero training.

His legacy? Picture this: a name that shines brighter than a basketball court under stadium lights. He was the Steve Jobs of basketball, always finding new tricks and using them to outsmart everyone else. He didn't just coach; he created a symphony of victory that echoed through the years.

So, young ballers, whenever you think of the magic of winning, remember Pat Riley. The silver-haired legend looked like he had a secret smile just for winning. Just like him, welcome change, believe in your magic, and shoot for the stars. Your basketball journey is a canvas waiting for your unique strokes of genius.

We don't know what life holds in store for us, but one thing is for sure. It changes. If you can move and bend with these changes and not battle them or try to hold onto

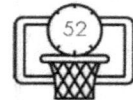

the past and how things used to be, you can do many amazing things just like Pat.

As you dribble through life, remember to share the magic of treating your sporting buddies well and with respect. Play hard, celebrate winning, and take on losing with the grace of a true champion. Pat Riley's legacy isn't just about basketball; it's about creating a world where everyone wins.

So, let the legend of Pat Riley be your playbook for greatness. With every dribble, every pass, every shot, and every change let his magic inspire you to be unstoppable, to become one who rises above others, and to leave a mark that changes the game.

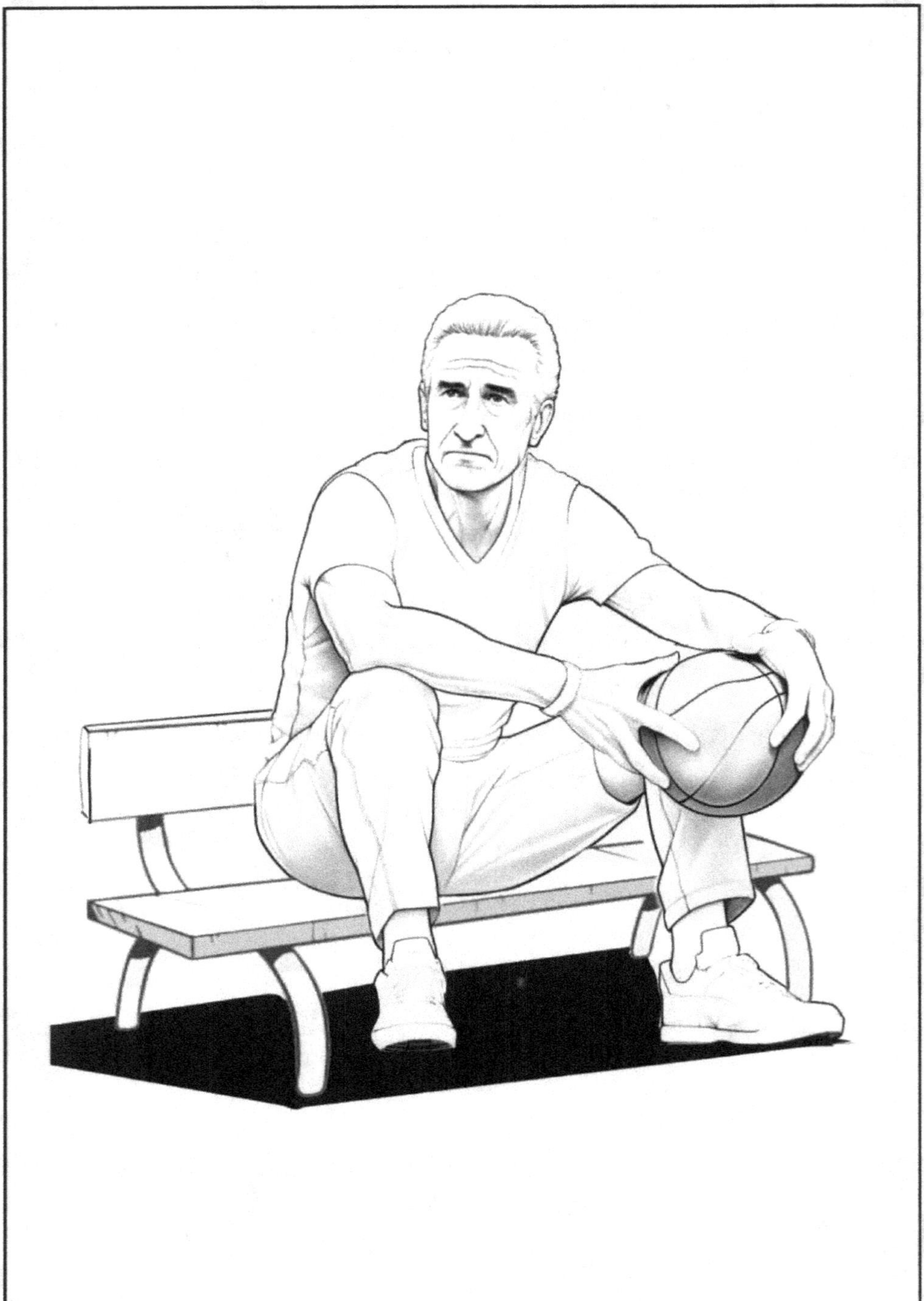

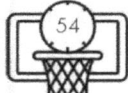

CHAPTER 10

SKY HIGH GLORY—LIZ CAMBAGE'S EPIC OLYMPIC DUNK

The crack of thunder roared across the stadium during an Olympic basketball game, and what happened next left everyone on their feet in total shock. In a show of pure athleticism, superhuman style, and crazy skill, one of the players soared through the air and landed a slam dunk that will go down in history as one of the greatest ever witnessed!

Meet Liz Cambage, the 6-foot-8 basketball superstar from Australia. She's not your ordinary player; she's a basketball giant with dreams as big as her height! And guess what? Liz made history with a jaw-dropping move that sent shockwaves through the stadium!

On that day, the stadium vibrated with excitement. Australia and Russia were neck-and-neck, both teams hungry for the win. Liz dribbled the ball toward the net—just one foot from winning—but she paused and leapt into the air like a gazelle in flight. With grace and ease, she soared and planted her hand around the edge of the backboard. Her teammates held their breath as she released her fingers from the rim—the swish, followed by a roar of cheers, signifying the perfect dunk. Every eye in the court was glued to Liz, who stood proudly at center court, basking in the glory of what she'd done.

People couldn't believe what they had just seen! Even her coach, Carrie Graf, was bursting with pride. She had encouraged Liz to practice dunking in warmups and seeing her do it in a real game was a dream come true. This is a moment, too, to see how important teamwork is, the huge impact of excellent coaches and the way they push their players to be their very best. In many cases, it's as if the coach has also scored that dunk.

But here's the funny part - Liz said she was always shy about dunking! Can you imagine that? Even with all her basketball talent, she felt a little shy about showing off her dunking skills. Well, guess what, Liz? You blew us all away, and now you're a basketball legend!

The best part of it all was how Liz's dunk spread happiness and excitement in the basketball world. People from all over the globe were talking about her historic move. It was like a basketball earthquake—shaking the sport and making it even more awesome!

So, kids, whenever you feel shy about something, remember Liz Cambage and her incredible dunk. She faced her fear and achieved something magical! She had decided at that moment, not to let her shyness get in the way of letting her talents shine. It's not showing off, it's more about letting your abilities bloom like a gorgeous flower. And it's a gift for others! It doesn't matter if you're shy or unsure; believe in yourself, work hard, and who knows? You might just create a moment that the world will remember forever! We should never hide our gifts!

Liz's dunk was more than just a point on the scoreboard; it was a symbol of girl power and basketball greatness. It showed that anyone, no matter their size or background, can achieve amazing things!

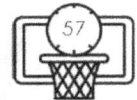

So, the next time you step on the basketball court, remember Liz Cambage's epic dunk and let it inspire you to reach for the stars. Who knows, maybe one day, you'll be the one making basketball history and bringing joy to fans all around the world.

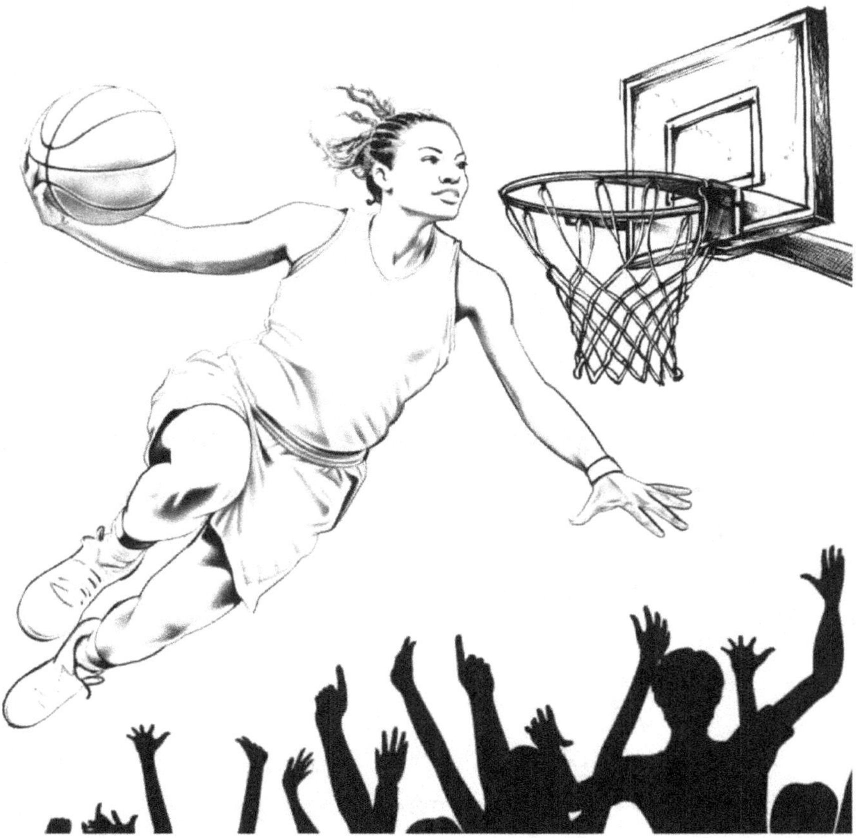

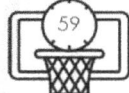

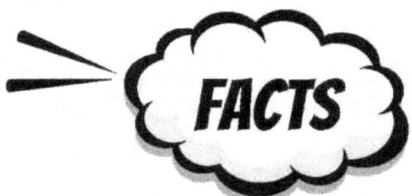

1. Basketball in the Olympics: Basketball has been a popular game at the Olympics since 1936 when it was first added.

2. Shot Clock: The shot clock came into play in 1954. It tells teams how long they must try a shot (24 seconds in the NBA and 30 seconds in college basketball) to keep the game moving quickly.

3. Basketball is popular all over the world. Millions of people worldwide play and love basketball, and leagues and events in places like Spain, China, and Argentina add to its global appeal.

4. Two-Basketball Game: A version of basketball called "Two-Basket Basketball" it has two hoops on the same court where teams contend. It is played at the same time with two balls.

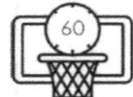

5. World's Largest Basketball: The Basketball Hall of Fame in Springfield, Massachusetts, has a huge basketball that is more than 30 feet across and weighs 10 tons.

CHAPTER 11

THE SUPERFAN—NAV'S INCREDIBLE JOURNEY

Get ready to step into the vibrant heart of Toronto, a place where the air is buzzing with basketball excitement! Among the sea of fans, there's one guy who shines like a superstar beacon—Nav Bhatia. With his unmistakable turban and beard, he's not just a fan; he's a living legend, a symbol of everything that makes basketball a thrilling adventure.

Now, let's take a jump back to the roaring '90s when the Toronto Raptors burst onto the scene. The city was buzzing with anticipation, and guess who was leading the fan department? That's right, Nav! He was like a human firework, lighting up the arena with his turbo-charged enthusiasm and energy. Boom!

Imagine this: at every home game, there's Nav, front and center, unleashing his superpower—the power of being the loudest, proudest, and most passionate fan. His trademark turban becomes a beacon of excitement, like a light in the dark! And his cheers ring through the air like thunderclaps. The energy he brings to the stands is like an invisible wave that flows through the crowd, and of course, gives energy to the other players on the court.

But here's where it gets even cooler. Nav's love for the game isn't just about pumping up the crowd; it's about making a difference. He's teamed up with the Raptors to spread the magic of basketball beyond the court's boundaries. Together, they're creating a whirlwind of positive vibes, inspiring kids, bringing communities together, and showing everyone that basketball isn't just a sport; it's a superpower of unity and fun! Of hanging out and enjoying each other's company.

The Raptors aren't just a team to Nav; they're family. But he's not just shouting for them; he's shouting for every dreamer, every kid with a passion, and every person who believes in the enchantment of basketball. His turbo-charged spirit isn't just about the cheers; it's about bringing

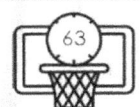

people together, creating memories, and celebrating the joy of the game.

So, to all you young ballers out there, let Nav Bhatia's story be your playbook. When you're on the court, dribbling with all of your might and aiming for that perfect shot, remember the guy who turned the stands into a roaring sea of excitement. Basketball isn't just about the scores; it's about the energy, the teamwork, and the unforgettable moments that make you feel alive.

Be a fan like Nav, not just in the arena, but in life. Spread the love, lift your teammates up, and show the world that basketball is a dance of passion and a song of being together. Nav has the Raptors, and you've got your own stage to shine on. So, dribble with joy, shoot with thrill, and let the basketball magic carry you to new heights!

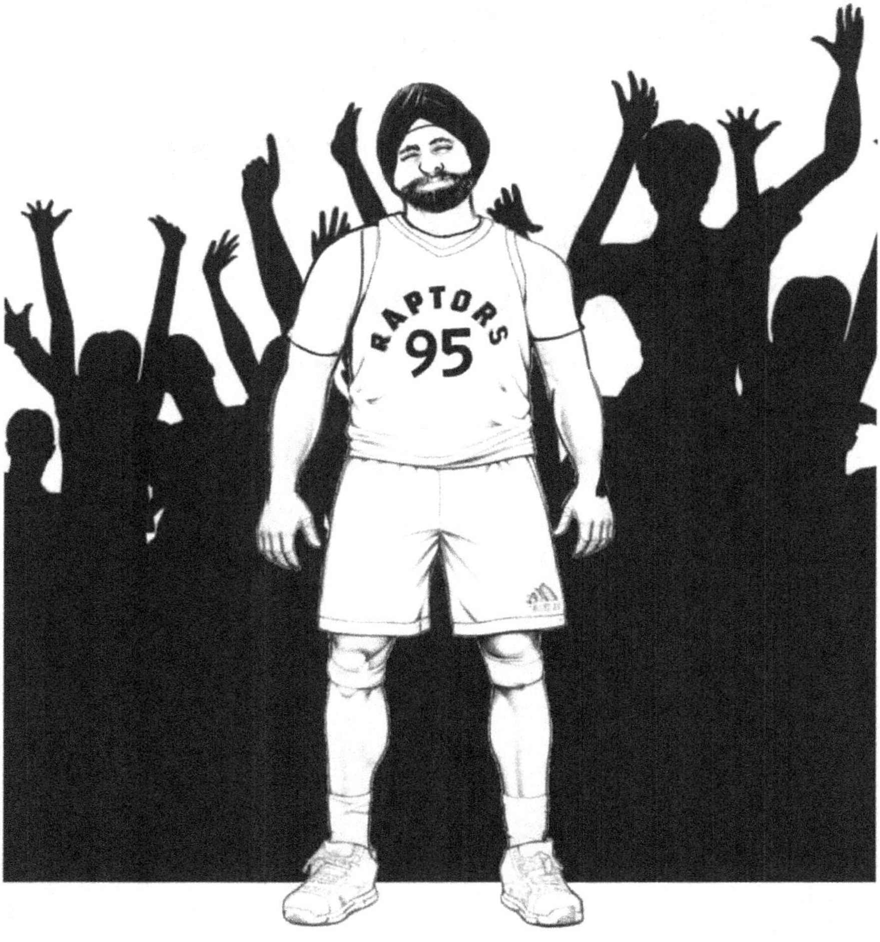

CHAPTER 12

BILL RUSSELL—THE GIANT GAME CHANGER WHO DUNKED ON INEQUALITY

We hope you're enjoying the incredible world of basketball, where giants roam the court, and scores light up the scoreboard. Let's now take a slam-dunk journey back in time to the early days of the game and meet a true game changer, the legendary Bill Russell!

Picture this: Basketball's early days were all about quick moves and speed, and taller players were considered too slow. But guess what? Along came Bill Russell, a towering force with a mind full of innovative ideas that would change the game forever.

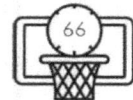

Back then, giants of the court were not the norm. Joe Lapchick, a star in the 1920s and 1930s, was only 6'5". Even in the late 1940s, a 6'10" player named George Mikan was powerful but a bit on the clunky side. Basketball was like a half-court dance, and different types of players were still making their way into the sport.

Now, enter Bill Russell. From his first championship with the University of San Francisco in 1955 to his Boston Celtics' triumphs in 1969, he wasn't just a player; he was a game changer on and off the court.

But let's rewind a bit. Born in Louisiana in the 1930s, Russell knew the struggles of life. His family moved to California to escape tough times, and while things were different and better in some ways, they weren't all smooth sailing. Russell faced many hard times and inequality, but he didn't back down.

Basketball wasn't his first love, but it became his ultimate passion. He brought a new kind of defense, jumping to block shots and causing chaos for opponents. Even when coaches didn't understand, Russell stuck to his guns, playing from the heart, and his new and unique way of playing became his superpower.

Fast forward to college. Russell joined the University of San Francisco, and with his towering height, he helped lead the team to NCAA titles. He changed the game with his aggressive style and was part of the first-ever college basketball team with three black starters.

Race wasn't just a game changer on the court; it was part of Russell's journey. He stood strong against racism, like when he and his teammates refused to play a game to protest discrimination. If things were unfair, he was sure to stand up for what was right and would not back down until changes were made. Russell showed that basketball was about more than just winning—it was about standing up for what's right.

As the NBA changed, so did Russell. Playing for the Celtics, he led his team to 11 championships in 13 years, taking on rival Wilt Chamberlain in epic battles. But Russell's impact wasn't just about his incredible skills; it was about his voice. He spoke out against racism, making his mark not only as a player but also as a champion for equality, and for things being fair for all players.

Through the civil rights movement and beyond, Russell stood tall as a light of change. He proved that athletes can be heroes off the court, using their voices to make a difference. Whether it was joining integrated basketball camps or speaking out against discrimination, he showed the world that basketball is more than just a game; it can be a stage for showing positive change.

So, young ballers, remember Bill Russell's story. Just like he transformed the game and stood up for what's right, you can be game changers in your own way. Enjoy and welcome diversity and all the different types of players you come across on the court, and off. Stand up against inequality, call it out! And when things are unfair, let your passion for basketball make even more positive changes in the world. As you dribble and shoot, remember that the real magic of the game isn't just in the points you score, but in the impact you make, both on and off the court.

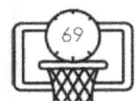

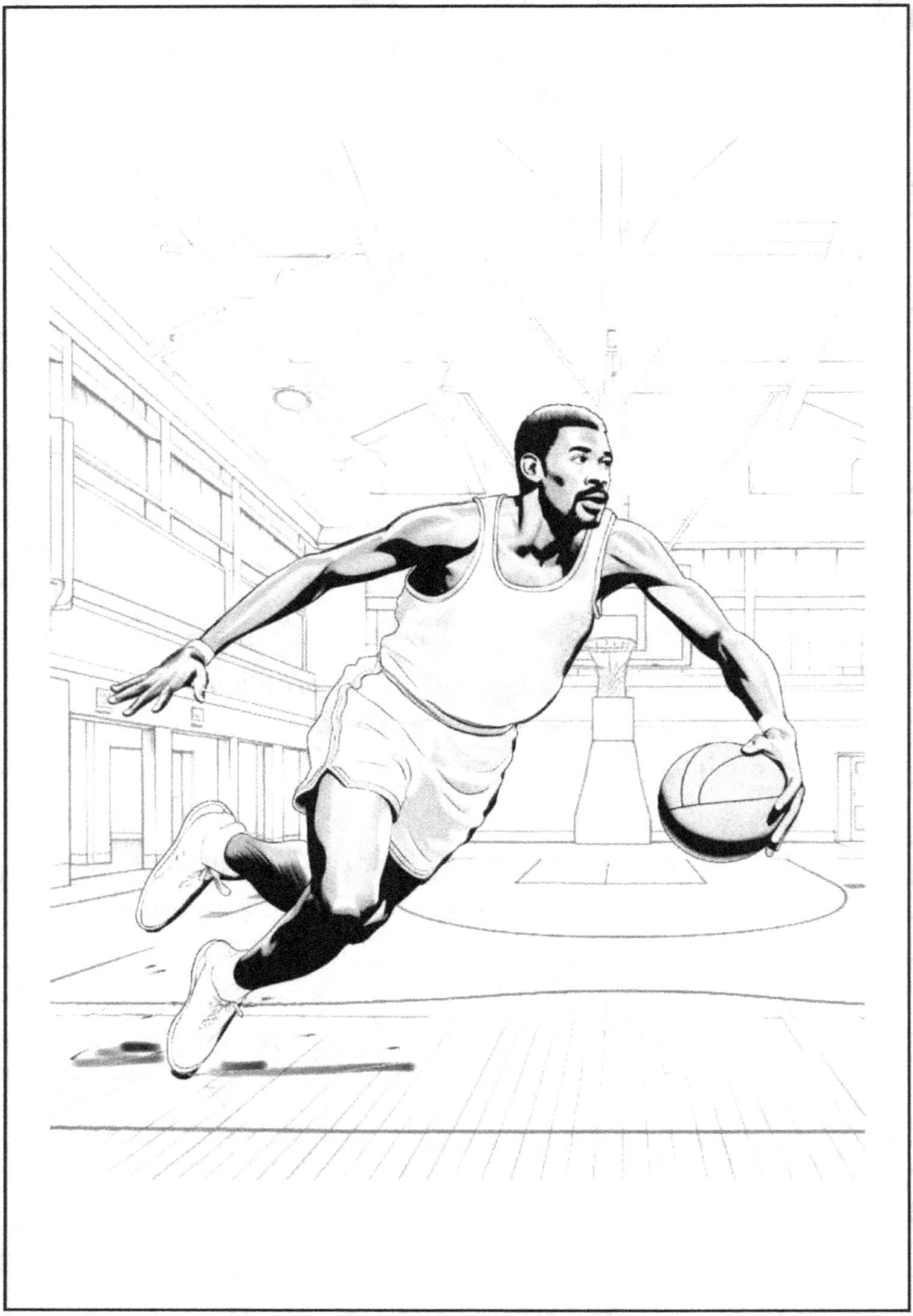

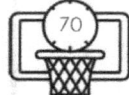

CHAPTER 13

SHOOTING FOR THE STARS

In the lively city of Kunming, China, where the sun painted the sky with the brightest of colors, an amazing story was told on a local basketball court. It was here that a young man named Luo Xiangjian showed the world that even with challenges, you could still reach for the stars and make magic happen.

Picture this: one sunny afternoon, when the air was filled with the sounds of laughter and the bouncing of basketballs, somebody walking by noticed something extraordinary. Something you just don't see every day! There, on the court, was Luo Xiangjian, a young man with an incredible spirit and a truly special gift. You see, despite having just one leg, he was dribbling, shooting, and making the most amazing three-point shots!

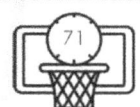

People couldn't believe their eyes. They stopped in their tracks to watch in shock and wonder as Luo's basketball soared through the net. His moves were so cool that someone decided to film him in action. Then, the video of Luo's incredible skills spread like wildfire on social media, capturing the hearts of kids and grown-ups all around the world.

But the story didn't start there. It actually began when Luo was just a little boy, five years old to be exact. Back then, he faced a big challenge—he lost his right leg because of an old, unexploded bomb. But even though life threw him a curveball, a big one, Luo's spirit stayed strong, and nothing could break it.

As Luo grew older, he found something that made his heart race with excitement—basketball! He just loved it! Every time he held a basketball and started dribbling, all his worries just disappeared. Like magic. He felt like he could do anything, and that the court was a place where dreams could come true. It made him forget all about his challenges.

But Luo wasn't so skilled from birth. He put the work in and practiced and practiced, sometimes spending hours and hours at the gym. He worked on his dribbling, perfected his shooting, and practiced his favorite move—the incredible three-point shot. With each shot that went in, Luo felt a burst of joy. He could see for himself the hard work paying off and knew then that with hard work, anything was possible.

And guess what? The more he practiced, the better he got and the more his confidence grew. He started really going for it and making shots that amazed everyone who saw them. Luo's spirit shone as brightly as the sun, and he wanted to share his joy with others.

Then came the moment that changed everything—the day Luo was seen playing at the local basketball court. The passerby was amazed by his incredible skills and his determination to keep going, even when things were tough. This passerby knew they had to share Luo's magic with the world, and that's how the viral video was born.

People from far and wide saw the video and cheered for Luo. They sent messages of support and encouragement, amazed by his positive attitude and determination. It

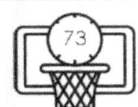

wasn't just about basketball skills; it was about showing that no challenge was too big to overcome, and if you love a sport, or anything for that matter, it can help you manage the hardest of struggles. It's all about finding what you love, what you're good at, and just going for it!

Luo's story became an inspiration to kids just like you. It showed that with passion, hard work, and a little bit of magic, you could achieve amazing things. Luo's journey wasn't always easy, but he never gave up. He kept practicing, believing in himself, and spreading happiness wherever he went.

And so, the story of Luo Xiangjian reminds us all to follow our dreams, just like he did on that local basketball court. Whether you're dribbling a basketball, drawing a picture, or learning something new, remember that with determination and a sprinkle of magic, you can make incredible things happen. Just like Luo, you have the power to reach for the stars and shine bright!

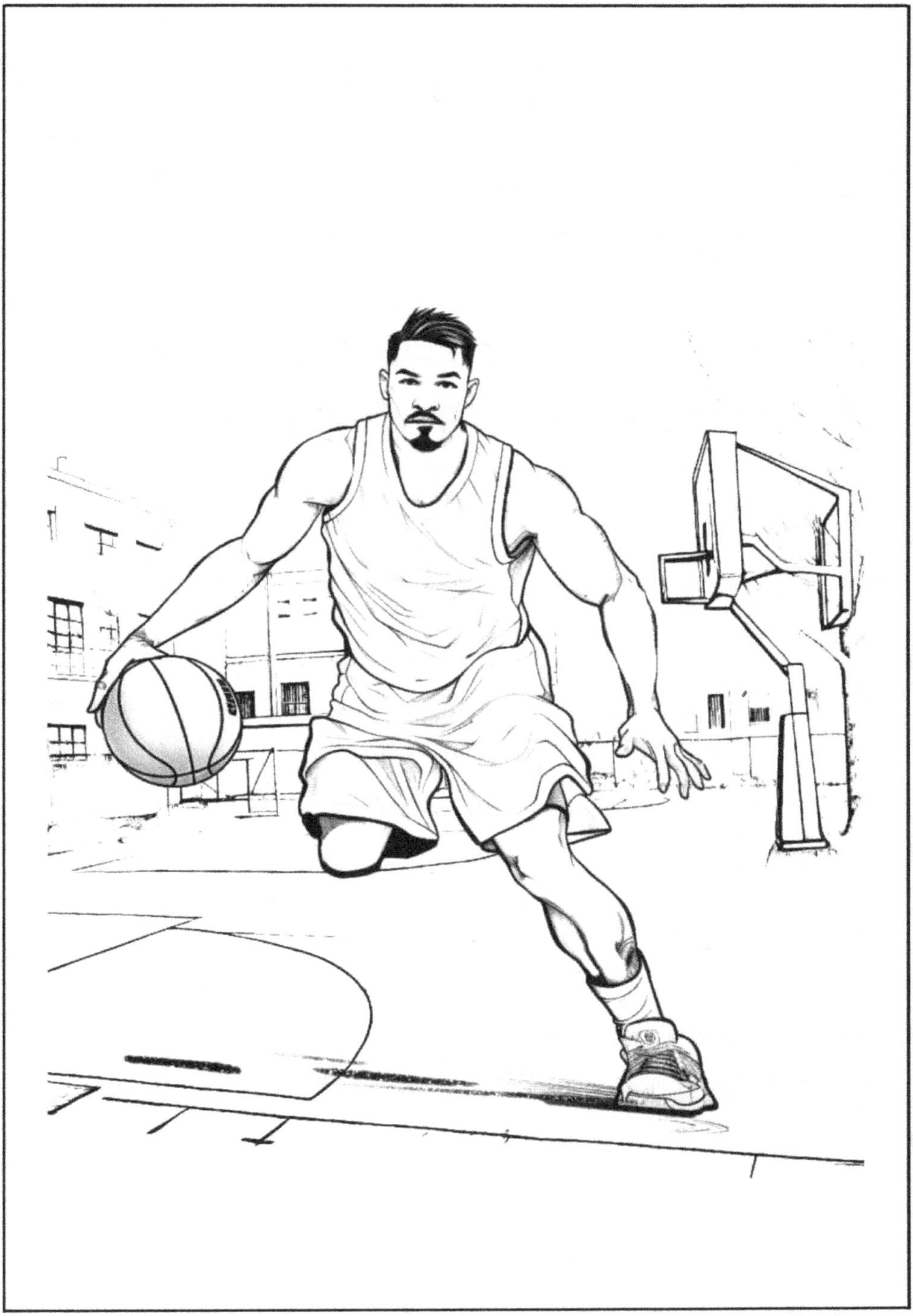

CHAPTER 14

THE UNSTOPPABLE J-MAC—A TRIUMPH OF DREAMS AND DETERMINATION

Many years ago, at Greece Athena High School, there was an extraordinary student named Jason McElwain, or J-Mac as his friends called him. J-Mac was autistic and had difficulty developing basic skills, such as not being able to speak until he turned five and not being able to chew food until he reached six. That must have been hard! He didn't let this stop him though, and instead he dedicated himself to something he loved; basketball, which became his life passion. See here again, how a passion for something can get you through the hardest of times.

When J-Mac reached high school, he practiced basketball day and night, dreaming of making the team. But he was still small, and he didn't quite make the cut. It must have been so upsetting for him seeing as he loved basketball so much. But don't worry, because the school gave him a special role as the student manager, so that he was still included in and he could be a part of his favorite game. Now, that's a teacher, who came up with this idea and we can learn something from this too – to include others the best we can. Because there's not much worse than feeling left out. And we can see that you don't need to be perfect at something to still enjoy it a lot!

J-Mac took his job super seriously, wearing a cool suit and tie to games, making sure he made it to every practice, and pretending like he was playing in the game. It was as close as he could get to playing, and instead of giving up, he made the best of it and loved being close to the action! The thing is, simply by watching and being so involved in the game, he would have learned a lot, and all of that got him closer to his dream. If he'd given up, he'd never have had all that enjoyment and opportunity.

For four years, J-Mac never stopped trying to play on the team, and he never lost his dedication. Four years! Then,

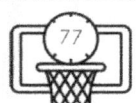

during the very last game of his senior year, something awesome happened. I bet you can guess! Yes, the coach surprised him with his own basketball jersey and gave him a chance to play in the game! Can you imagine his excitement?

When J-Mac got onto the court, he missed the first two shots he took, but that didn't slow him down. Instead, he upped his game, kept his focus and suddenly turned into a basketball superstar! In the last four minutes of the game, J-Mac scored an incredible 20 points! The entire school erupted with excitement, cheering and celebrating this unforgettable moment. And to think if he let those first few missed shots make him give up!

J-Mac's heartwarming and inspiring story spread all over the country! He won awesome awards like the ESPY award for Best Moment in Sports and the Teen Choice Courage Award. He even got to meet famous athletes like Peyton Manning and Magic Johnson! J-Mac became a shining example of never giving up on your dream, making the very best of situations, and overcoming obstacles. And he's still inspiring kiddies by featuring in this book! Too cool, right?

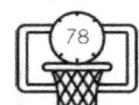

Remember J-Mac's fantastic journey. It will remind you that no matter what challenges come your way, with hard work, dedication, and never giving up, you can achieve amazing things! Let's all be like J-Mac, shining stars who conquer every game of life with a big smile!

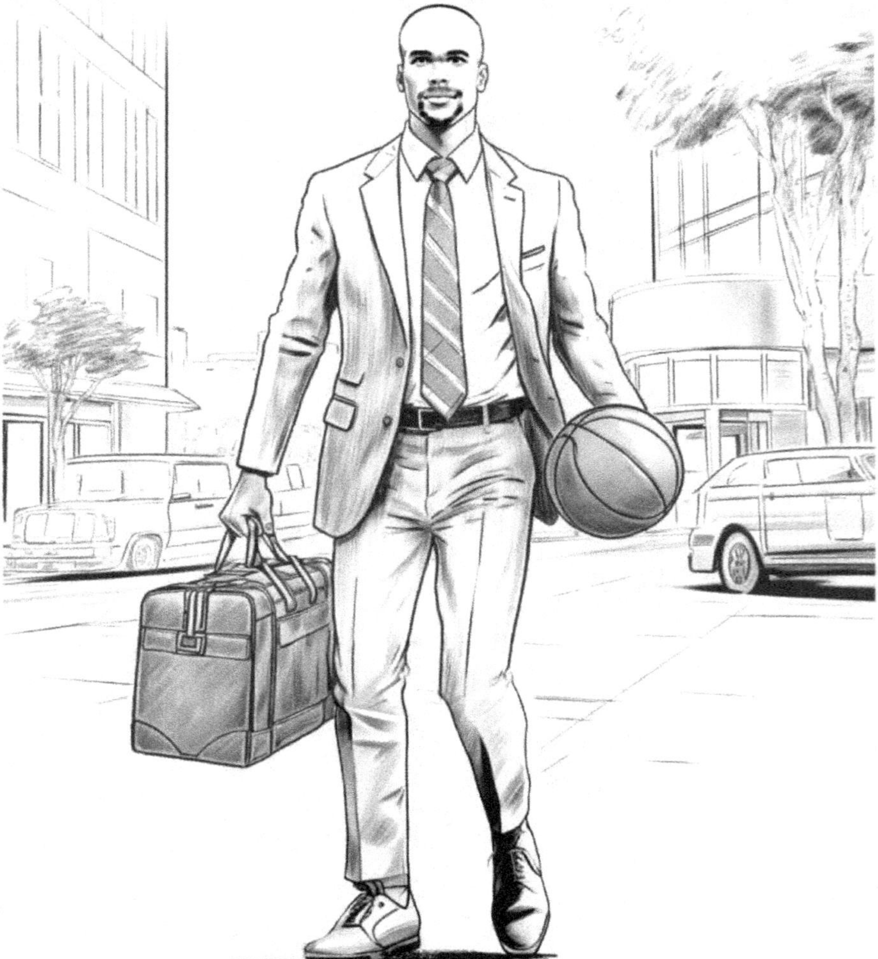

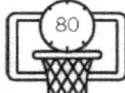

CHAPTER 15

FROM ROOKIE TO CHAMP— MAGIC'S MEGA VICTORY!

Step into the time machine, my young friends, and let me whisk you back to the dazzling year of 1980. The NBA Finals were rocking the basketball world like a groovy dance party! The Los Angeles Lakers were squaring off against the Philadelphia 76ers in a showdown that had fans everywhere glued to their seats.

Now, let me set the stage for you. It's Game 6, and the Lakers are ahead in the series. But hold on to your basketballs because guess what? The Lakers' towering star, Kareem Abdul-Jabbar, was resting a sprained ankle and chillaxing back in Los Angeles. Oh no, right? But wait, who's that bursting onto the scene? It's none other than the rookie sensation, Earvin "Magic" Johnson!

Get this: Magic wasn't just your average rookie. Nope, he was like a basketball magician with a hat full of tricks! And guess what? In this epic showdown, he decided to take on ALL the positions! I mean, who does that? Only someone as magical as Magic Johnson, that's who!

Imagine this: the crowd is roaring, the tension is thicker than peanut butter, and Magic is zipping around the court like a blur of awesomeness. He's like a one-man circus, dribbling, passing, and shooting like nobody's business. The fans are going bananas, wondering if they've been transported to a wacky, different basketball universe.

But wait, there's more! Magic's skills were on display like a fireworks show on the Fourth of July. He scores an unbelievable 42 points—seriously, 42! He grabs 15 rebounds, like he's plucking oranges off a tree, and to top it all off, he serves up seven assists with a side of basketball magic sauce. Can you believe it? It's like he's playing a video game with cheat codes! He sure was on fire.

And hold onto your basketball shorts, because the Lakers didn't just win the game, they won it in style with a score of 123-107! Magic's enchanting performance was like a

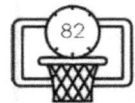

clever trick that turned the Lakers into champions, and the crowd erupted in cheers, confetti, and probably a few moonwalks.

But here's the cherry on top of this basketball sundae: Magic Johnson wasn't just a baller on the court. Oh no, he was also a superstar off the court, lighting up the world with his megawatt personality! Can you believe that while the Lakers were jetting from Los Angeles to Philadelphia, Magic, with his mischievous grin, decided to claim Kareem's seat? He winked at the coach and declared, "Never fear, E.J. is here!" Can you imagine the coach's jaw dropping to the floor?

Magic Johnson wasn't just a name; it was a guarantee of excitement! The basketball court and the spotlight were like his best buddies, and together, they created comedy gold that no one could resist. He made the very best of his stardom and the opportunities that brought and shared it with the world around him.

So, my fellow adventurers in the land of hoop dreams, remember this tale of Magic Johnson. When life throws you a curveball, be ready to step up to the plate and hit

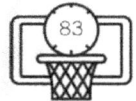

a home run of awesomeness! Whether you're a rookie or a seasoned player, let your personality shine like a disco ball, and who knows, you might just conjure up some magic of your own. So, embrace challenges with a grin as wide as Magic's and dance your way to winning on the court of life. You're the real MVP of your own story!

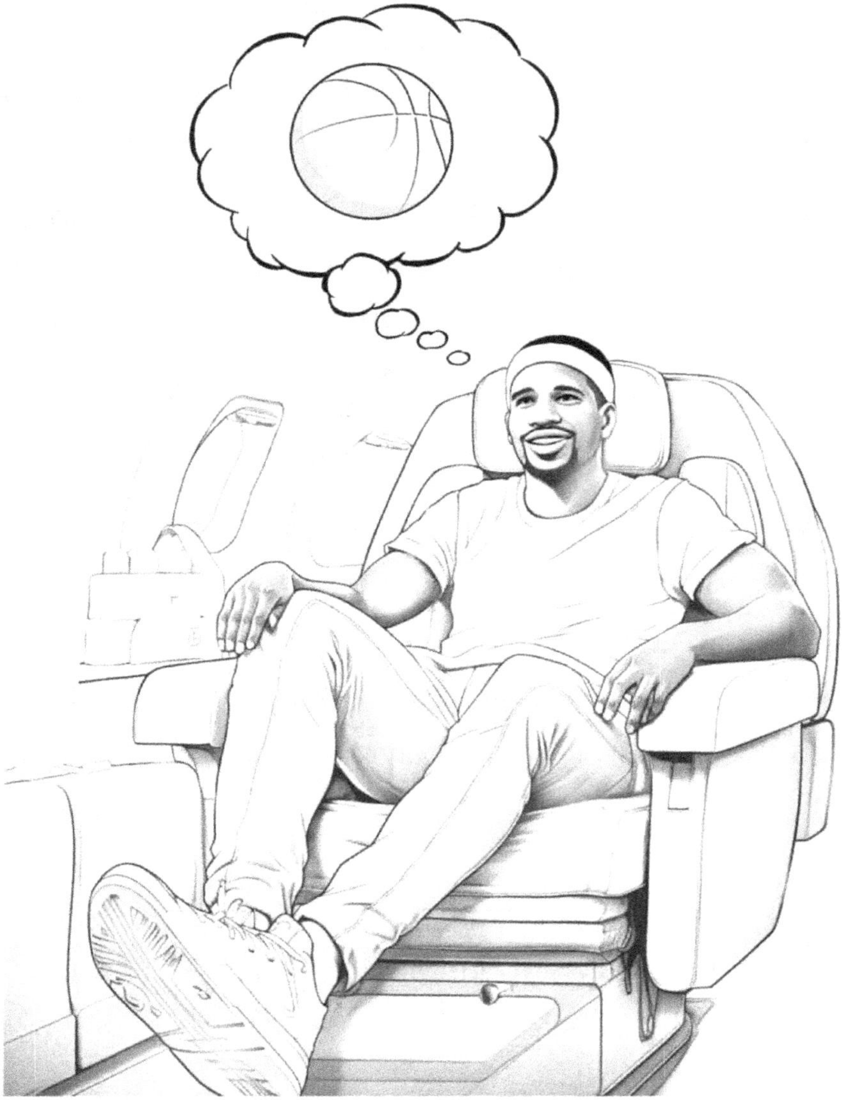

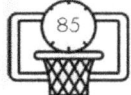

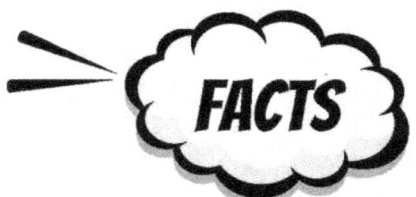

1. Basketball and the White House: To help him relax and stay in shape during World War 2, President Franklin D. Roosevelt had a secret basketball court built in the White House.

2. Basketball Robot: In Japan, a robot called "CUE" was made that can shoot basketballs with great accuracy and make almost all of the shots it takes.

3. A comparison of court sizes: An NBA basketball court is so big that you could fit almost three of them on an NFL football field.

4. Longest Basketball Game: The longest basketball game ever recorded went on for 76 hours and 20 minutes. That's more than three days of basketball games that never stop.

5. Half-Court Shots: The furthest half-court shot ever made in a basketball game was from 89 feet away! It's the same as getting a goal from the other end of the court.

CHAPTER 16

THE HICK FROM FRENCH LICK— LARRY BIRD'S LEFT-HANDED GAME

Get ready to be transported back to a basketball time filled with wild tales and jaw-dropping skills! We're diving into the world of Larry Bird, the Hick from French Lick, where the hardwood court became his stage for some unforgettable basketball magic.

Here's the deal: it's Valentine's Day in the year 1986, and Larry Bird is ready to sprinkle some enchantment onto the basketball court. But he's not planning for just any ordinary game—oh no! Larry is about to pull off a left-handed extravaganza against the super-tough Portland Trail Blazers. Hold onto your basketball jerseys, and forget your chocolates and roses, because this game is about to get wild!

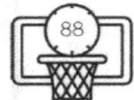

Now, let's set the scene. The game is hanging in the balance, the tension is thick enough to cut with a basketball. And what does Larry decide to do? With a wink and a grin, he surprises everyone with a spur-of-the-moment decision: he's going to dominate the court with his non-dominant hand—his left hand! Can you even fathom dribbling, passing, and shooting with your opposite hand? It's like a basketball comedy show! So tricky! Have a go and try it out it!

Larry Bird transformed into a true basketball trickster. It's like his left hand was sprinkled with fairy dust! He scored an astronomical 47 points, snatched 14 rebounds out of thin air, served up 11 assists like they were on a silver platter, snagged the ball away from opponents, and oh, did I mention he even blocked two shots? This was a stat line that defies the laws of basketball physics!

Hold onto your headbands because it gets even crazier. Out of the 34 field goal attempts Larry made, a whopping 10 were with his left hand! And here's the jaw-dropper: he didn't miss a single free throw, going a perfect 7-of-7 from the line. It's like his left hand had a magical spell that made every shot find its mark!

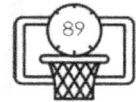

Now, brace yourselves for the punchline that had everyone in stitches. When the game ended, the media swarmed Larry, curious about his daring left-handed spree. They just had to know all the details! And do you know what he told them, flashing that trademark Larry Bird grin? He said, "I'm saving my right hand for the Lakers!" That's right, he had some special tricks up his sleeve for the showdown with the Los Angeles Lakers! What a cool comment!

But the magic didn't stop there, my friends. Just two days after the Portland game, the Boston Celtics faced off against their arch-nemeses, the Los Angeles Lakers. And what happened? You guessed it, they won again! Larry Bird swooped in, scoring 22 points, snatching 18 rebounds like they were hidden treasures, and dishing out 7 assists as if he had eyes in the back of his head. The court was practically on fire from all the sparks flying off his sneakers!

So, my fellow ballers-in-training, what's the lesson here? Let loose, have a blast, and be as daring as Larry Bird himself! Basketball is not just about making baskets; it's about unleashing your creativity and leaving everyone in shock with your magical moves. It's about trying something new and knowing that even if no one else has done it, it doesn't mean it's wrong, or can't be done, it absolutely

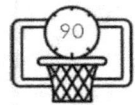

can! And if it's not against the rules, give it a whirl, you might just discover something new. At the very least, you'll have fun while you're at it and mix things up for the crowd. You might even make a headline or two. Be willing to step out of your comfort zone and surprise everyone because who knows? You might just conjure up some legendary basketball spells of your own, becoming the stuff of basketball folklore like the one and only Hick from French Lick!

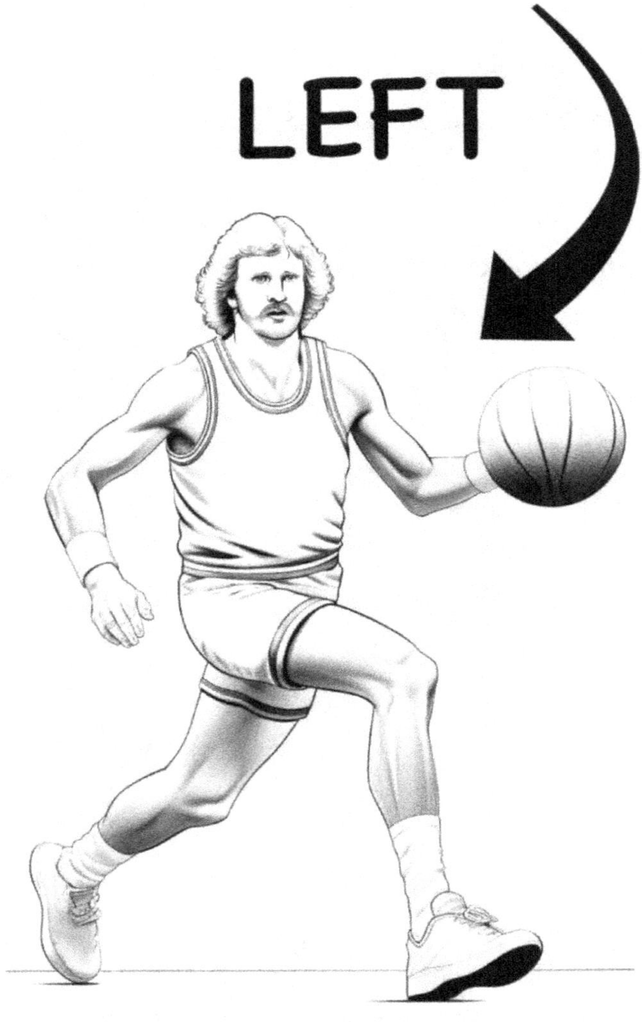

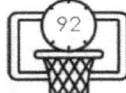

CHAPTER 17

LINSANITY UNLEASHED

Come one, come all! Let's journey back to the crazy year of 2012, where the city that never sleeps, New York City, was buzzing with the extraordinary tale of none other than Jeremy Lin, the basketball sensation making waves with the Knicks. Buckle up, because this story is about to take you on a ride full of unexpected twists and turns!

Imagine it: the Knicks were on a winning streak, and guess who was at the center of it all? You got it—Jeremy Lin, the young basketball prodigy who was causing a hoopla like never before. The fans were head over heels, chanting, "We want Lin!" It was as if they had discovered a treasure trove of basketball stardust and couldn't wait to see him shine on the court!

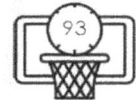

Now, here's the kicker: Jeremy Lin was just a sprightly 23-year-old! Yet, in the blink of an eye, he skyrocketed to celebrity status, capturing hearts across the globe. What made his story so interesting? So headline-worthy? Well, it was a tale of overcoming challenges with a dash of Hogwarts-level wizardry. After high school, he didn't nab a scholarship, but did he throw in the towel? Nope! He rolled up his sleeves, studied hard, and made his way to Harvard, proving that he was no ordinary player—he was equipped with magical skills!

But wait, there's more. The NBA draft rolled around, and you'd think every team would be racing to grab Jeremy, right? Well, the story took a twist—no teams picked him at first. What?! Now that would have been super disappointing. Did he give up? Absolutely not! He kept his chin up, pushed forward, and guess where he landed? You guessed it, the Knicks! Amazing. In a flash, he transformed into a basketball sensation, dazzling the world with a show that was more magical than a unicorn's dance routine! Have you seen a unicorn's dance routine? Well, it's pretty magical!

Jeremy's performances were like watching shock after wonderful shock, all played out on the grand stage of the basketball court. He moved with a grace that defied the

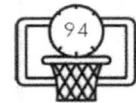

laws of physics, mixing sports, culture, and religion with a magic touch that left everyone spellbound. His journey hit the people deeply, especially with Asian-Americans who saw in him a true role model, blazing a trail of inspiration for other Asian Americans with big dreams of their own.

Even A-list celebrities like Spike Lee and Whoopi Goldberg couldn't resist the wonder of Jeremy's game. They watched, jaws dropped and eyes wide, as he unleashed a spellbinding display of moves and skills that were, well, out of this world!

But here's the secret ingredient to Jeremy's magic potion: he stayed as humble as a wizard living in a cupboard under the stairs. Amidst all the fame and spotlight, he remained true to himself, like a true magical hero.

So, here's the golden nugget of wisdom from Jeremy Lin's spellbinding story—always have faith in yourself, and never, ever let go of your dreams. No matter how tough the dungeon of challenges may seem, keep fighting, keep believing, and keep pushing forward. You've got superstar magic within you, and with every step of your magical journey, you'll inspire others and create a story

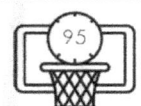

that's more enchanting than a fairy tale. Don't wait for your dreams to come true, go out and grab them!

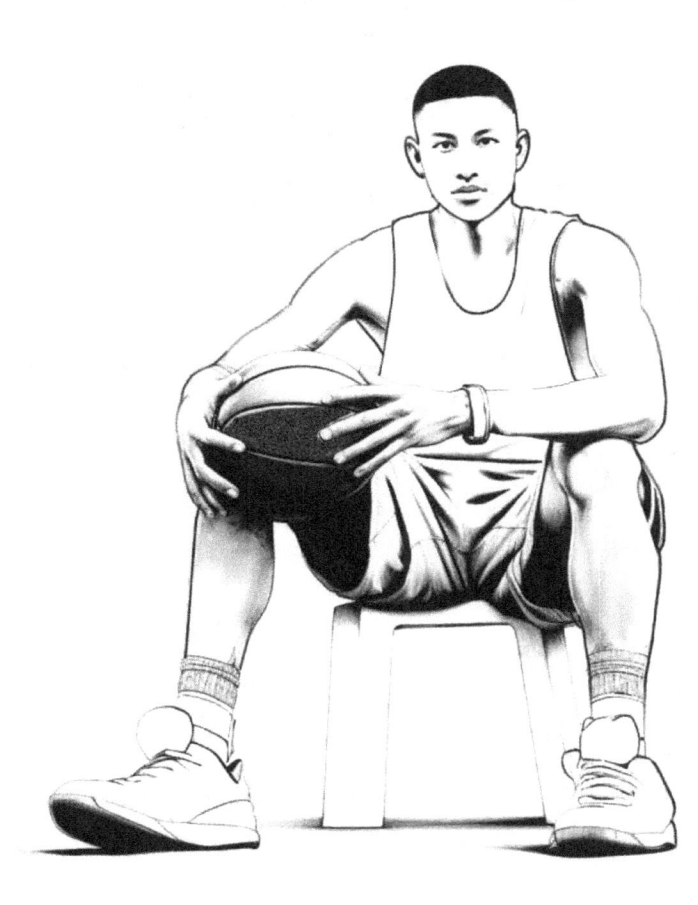

CHAPTER 18

MO CHEEK'S MOST MEMORABLE ASSIST

In the annals of the NBA, Maurice Cheeks was a brilliant player! And, after retiring from the court, he became an equally gifted coach, giving so much to the game. He also dedicated himself to important plans away from basketball.

As a player, Maurice was a superstar point guard who dished out more than 7,000 assists! But one of his biggest assists came when he was coaching the Portland Trail Blazers. There was a 13-year-old girl named Natalie Gilbert, who won a contest to sing the national anthem before a game. But she got nervous and forgot the words. Poor thing!

Guess what? Coach Cheeks to the rescue! He saw Natalie struggling and went right up to her, putting his arm around her, and helped her remember the words. Together, they finished the anthem, and the crowd cheered for both of them! What a legend. That's a real star, don't you think? He didn't just watch on, feeling sorry for the girl, he decided to do something about it, and what a difference it made for that little girl.

Maurice Cheeks was clearly not just a great coach but also a caring person who couldn't help but help others. He also loved his team, the Philadelphia 76ers deeply, and his hometown, Philadelphia. Even when he faced challenges as a coach, he always put in his best effort, not just for himself but for others.

Sometimes, things didn't go as planned, and that's life. It happens to us all at some time or another. He got fired from a coaching job. Sure, it would have been very disappointing, but that didn't stop Maurice from focusing on moving forward and being a true leader! He later coached the Detroit Pistons too, and he always gave his all.

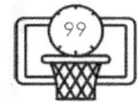

In 2018, Coach Cheeks was recognized for all his greatness on and off the court and was inducted into the Naismith Memorial Basketball Hall of Fame! It was a well-deserved honor for this incredible coach and person. Now, that's a life well lived.

The big lesson from Coach Maurice Cheeks's story is to be kind and help others when they need it. It can feel great to shoot some cool shots and to win games, but the feeling of helping someone else, of bringing a smile to their face can make you feel not just as great, but even better. Nothing beats those warm feelings in your heart when you know you did good for someone else. Just like he assisted Natalie, you can make a difference by being there for someone in their time of need. And no matter what challenges come your way, always give your best and never stop believing in yourself! One day, people might be recognizing you in some kind of Hall of Fame, too! We don't always need to be recognized though, do we? The feeling we have in our hearts from being kind or helping others can stay with us forever, and no one can take that away from us.

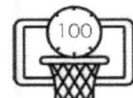

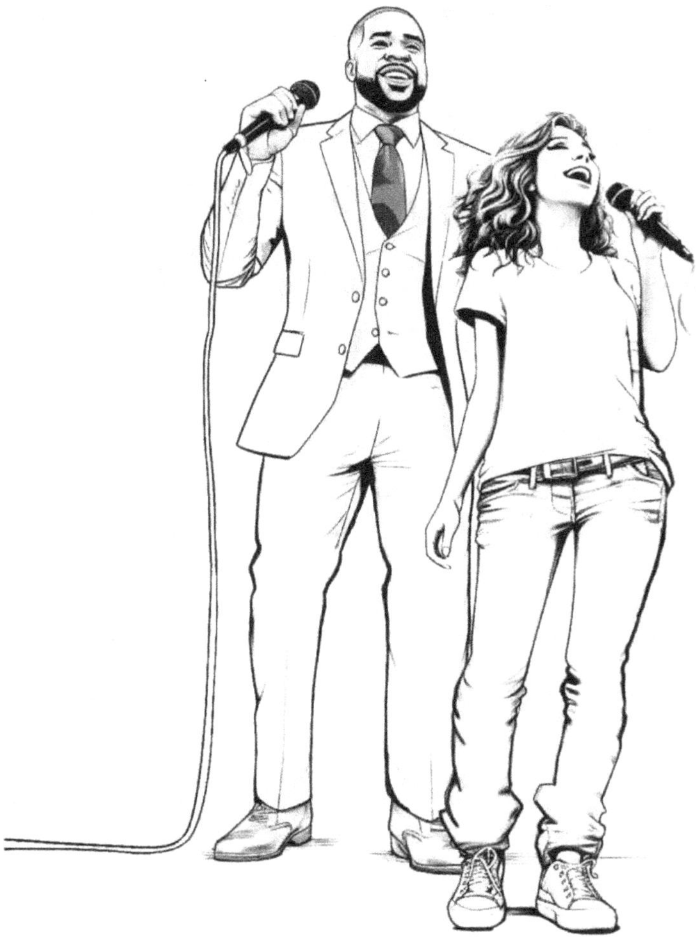

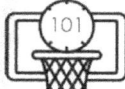

CHAPTER 19

ALONZO MOURNING'S COMEBACK—A TALE OF COURAGE AND TRIUMPH IN BASKETBALL

In the wild world of basketball, there was a superstar named Alonzo Mourning who spun his way through victories and challenges like a basketball whirlwind. But wait, there's a twist in this tale that you won't see coming! Alonzo was the king of the court, especially in his role as a center. He was so good that they even put his name in the Hall of Fame hallways. But just when everything seemed perfect, life threw a curveball his way—a kidney problem that made playing basketball feel like walking on a tightrope made of spaghetti. Sounds difficult? Well, it was!

So, let's rewind to before the 2000–01 season. Imagine Alonzo getting ready to rule the court like a basketball

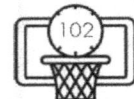

champ. But, uh-oh, here comes the tricky part—the kidney disease decides to join the game too. It puts a spell on Alonzo's skills, making it tough for him to play the way he used to. Talk about a challenge, right? It's like playing basketball with your shoelaces tied together and walking a tightrope of spaghetti!

Now, here's where the plot gets twistier than a pretzel. Alonzo decided to show the kidney disease who's boss. He did something super brave—he waved goodbye to the basketball court earlier than he planned. It was like retiring from a race while wearing roller skates! He just was not ready to slow down, but he knew he had to. Why, you ask? Well, his body needed a timeout from all the basketball action so that it could recover. If he pushed himself too far, he may have caused some permanent damage to his body. It was good he knew his limits and when to stop and rest.

But guess what? Our hero wasn't one to stay down for long. His cousin turned into his sidekick and brought a magical gift—a kidney transplant! With his cousin's superpower kidney and a ton of hard work, Alonzo made an epic comeback in less time than it takes to learn your ABCs!

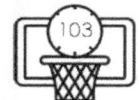

People everywhere couldn't believe their eyes. Alonzo was back on the court, showing off his basketball skills like a superhero showing off their cape! He joined the Nets, proving that no enemy—not even kidney disease—could keep him away from the game he loved. Can you imagine dribbling a basketball with one hand and holding a shield with the other? That's Alonzo for you: the basketball Avenger!

But wait, the games not over yet. Alonzo's journey was more exciting than a rollercoaster ride with a twist! He didn't just stop at his comeback; he played for four more seasons. And here's the slam dunk part—in 2005–06, he helped the Miami Heat win an NBA title! It's like scoring the winning goal while wearing a cape and juggling basketballs!

So, what's the magical lesson from Alonzo's basketball adventure? Never give up, even when things get trickier than solving a puzzle with your eyes closed. Alonzo faced challenges, but he tackled them with the heart of a lion and the skills of a basketball wizard. His journey teaches us to believe in ourselves, work hard, and never back down, no matter how tricky the court may seem. He also shows

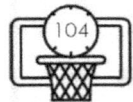

us how important rest is, and after a break, we can come back better than ever.

So, young ballers, let Alonzo Mourning's story be your secret potion of courage. If you face tough times, remember—just like Alonzo, you can rise like a phoenix and beat challenges with a basketball-sized smile. Play your game, chase your dreams, and remember, with a little magic in your heart, anything is possible!

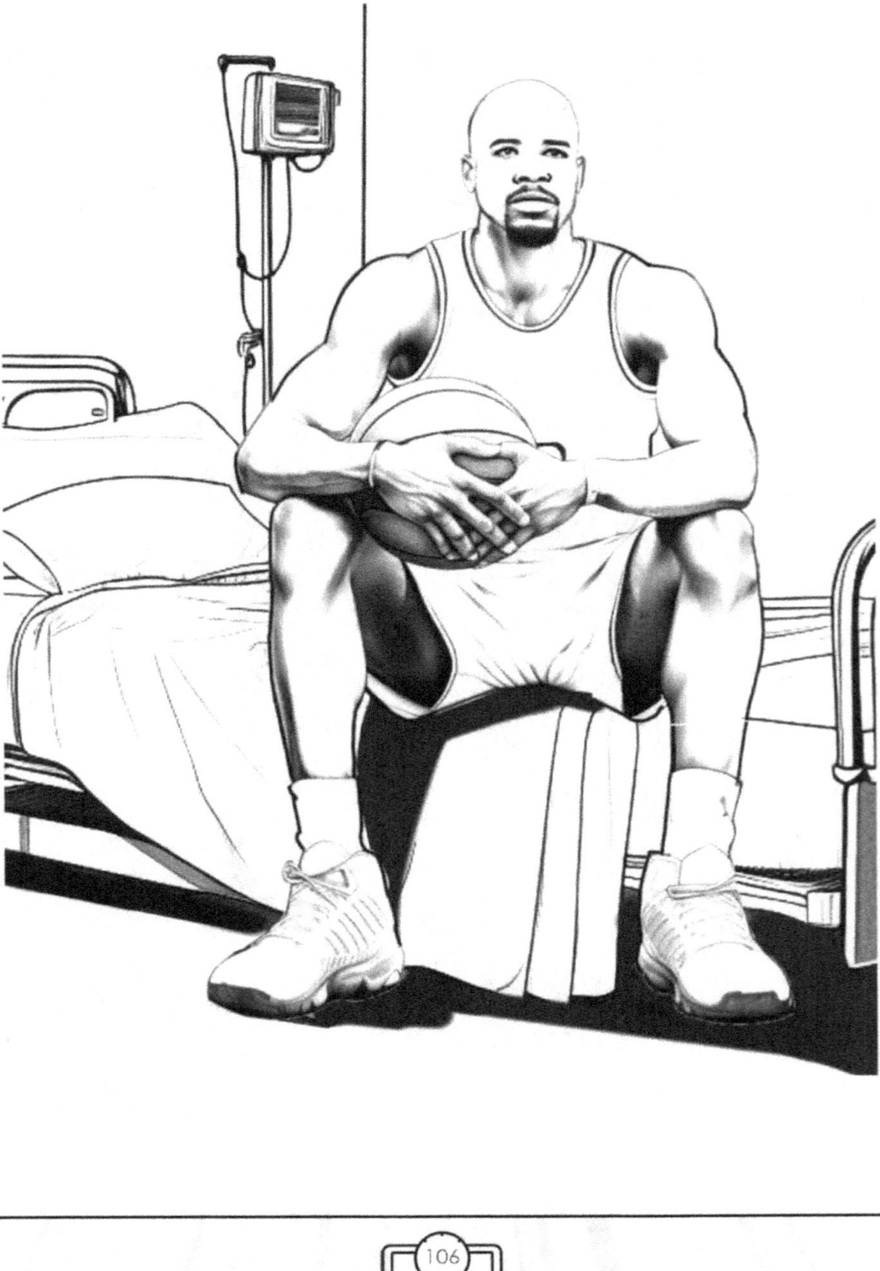

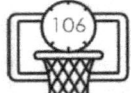

CHAPTER 20

THE SNEAKY SHOT HEARD 'ROUND THE COURT

I have a tale that'll have you laughing like a basketball bouncing down the court! It all went down during a Pelicans basketball game, the kind of day when magic seems to sneak its way onto the court. So, let me set the stage for you—players practicing their moves, fans roaring with excitement, and in the middle of it all, a super-daring fan cooking up a plan that's wilder than a slam dunk from half-court!

This brave person, let's call him Game-time Greg, decided to take fan engagement to a whole new level. Dressed in full Pelicans team gear, he made sure to blend right in with the real players. It was like he wanted to become part of the team's secret sauce, even if it was just for a brief, exhilarating moment.

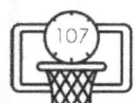

Now, here's where the magic happens. During the pre-game warm-ups, when everyone's eyes are glued to the court, Game-time Greg makes his move. He sneakily slips away from his seat, and guess what he does? He starts stretching and doing warm-up exercises right next to the actual players! Can you believe it? He is like a chameleon blending in with a bunch of flamingos. Nobody noticed a thing! It was like he had a superpower that made him invisible to basketball radars! A pretty cool invisibility cloak! Go, Greg! I bet his buddies were laughing their heads off.

But the story gets even funnier, my friends. The best bit was when Game-time Greg finally got his hands on the basketball. I know, it's hard to believe! Then, He mustered all his courage, aimed for the basket, and… oh dear, the ball missed the target by a mile! Boy, did he give it his best shot, though! It was like the ball had its own set of wings and decided to fly away! Oopsie Daisy, that was a miss! But you know what? It was a miss that turned into a hilarious slam dunk of laughter. Talk about some fun entertainment for the crowd. It was their lucky day!

And that's when the magic bubble burst—it became clear that Game-time Greg wasn't actually part of the team. For no one on the team would play that badly!

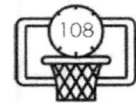

Security swooped in like basketball referees making sure the game's played fair and square. But guess what? Game-time Greg wasn't feeling down in the dumps. Oh no, he was beaming with joy! Why, you ask? Because he had just lived his basketball dream, even if it was just for a blink-and-you-miss-it moment. A memory to treasure forever! I bet he's told this story more than a few times, too!

Now, let's dive into the mystery within the magic—who was the secret passer of the ball to Game-time Greg? Was it a confused ball boy, caught in the whirlwind of the moment? Or did a real player give him the ball, thinking he was part of the team's secret playbook? Oopsie! It's a mystery that tickles the funny bone and adds a sprinkle of hilarity to this adventure on the court.

So, my fellow basketball fans, tuck this hilarious tale of Game-time Greg, the basketball ninja into your treasure chest of stories. It's a reminder that dreaming big and having a laugh is all part of the game. But, and here's the hoop you should never miss, always play by the rules, appreciate the game from the right seats, and enjoy the magic from the sidelines. It's not fair to interrupt the game like that. But who knows, one day you might have your very own remarkable basketball adventure that'll have

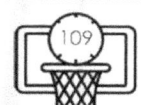

everyone cheering for you, without breaking the rules! As you've seen from all the stories you've read so far, it truly is possible!

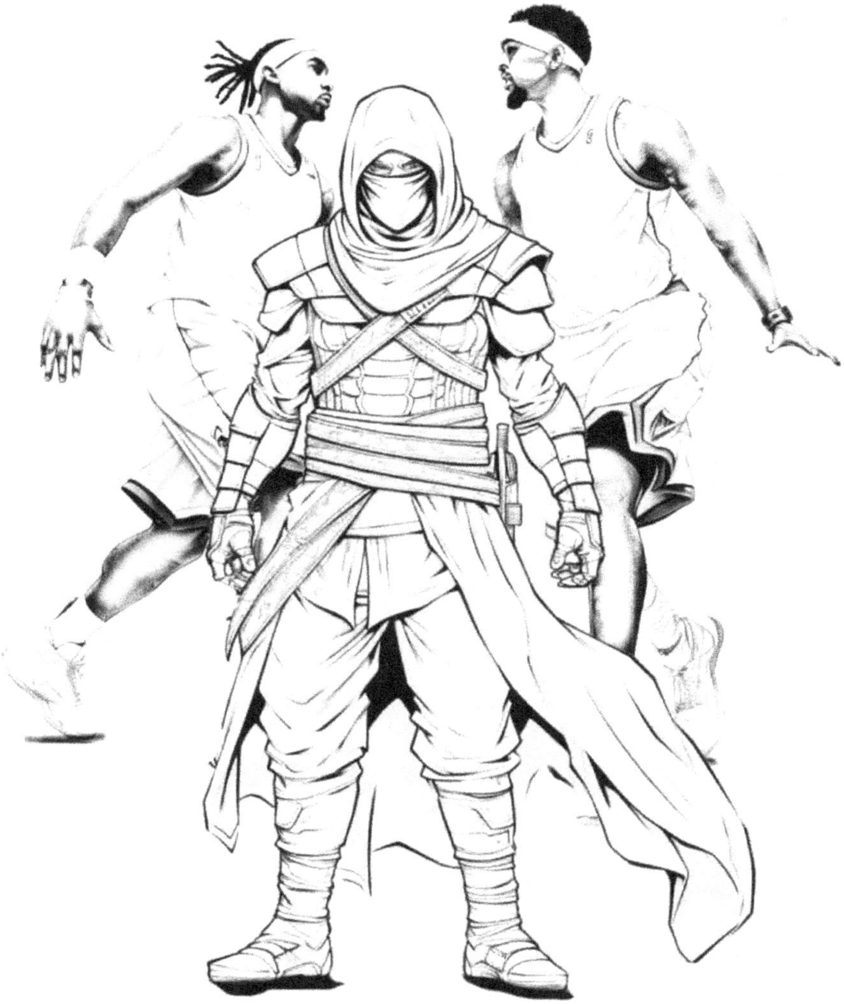

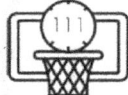

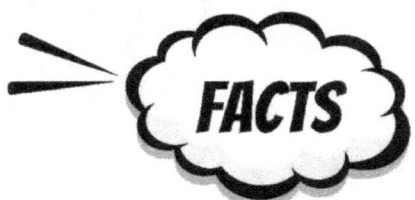

1. The Spalding Basketball Plant: Almost every NBA basketball used in games is made in a single plant in the small town of Chicopee, Massachusetts.

2. Rules about dribbling: Dribbling was not allowed in the early days of basketball. To move the ball down the court, players had to pass it to each other. Later, dribbling became a real part of the game.

3. Shaquille O'Neal's Shoe Size: The former NBA star wore a size 22 shoe. That's about twice as big as the average shoe size for an adult.

4. Wilt Chamberlain's 100-Point Game: In 1962, Wilt Chamberlain set an NBA record by scoring 100 points in a single game.

5. Most Basketball Bounces in One Minute: 872 basketball bounces in one minute is the best. In just 60 seconds, that's a lot!

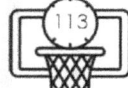

CONCLUSION

We hope you loved reading these fascinating tales as you've journeyed into the world of basketball. These stories are filled with instances of strength, tenacity, and a hint of the miraculous.

From the determined young athlete, Jeremy Lin, who defied all odds and won hearts worldwide with his "Linsanity," to the unstoppable spirit of Alonzo Mourning, who fought bravely the challenges of kidney disease and soared to new heights of success; we hope these stories have touched your hearts and inspired you to go after your own dreams.

Through the laughter and cheers, we witnessed Bango, the lovable mascot, turning a basketball game into a wild and hilarious adventure. He showed us that even in moments of fun and excitement, accidents can happen, but it's how we react to them that truly matters.

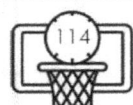

The story of the mystery fan, blending in with the Pelicans players, reminds us of the joy of imagination and daring to dream big. While we may not become basketball ninjas, we can unleash our creativity and embrace the magic of childhood wonder in our lives.

These inspiring tales teach us valuable life lessons. They remind us to believe in ourselves, overcome challenges, and embrace our unique journey. Like the fan who got his warm-up shot, we may face moments of being unsure, but it's how we bounce back that shapes our futures. No matter the obstacle, we can rise to new heights with determination and resilience just like the stars we admire.

So, as you embark on your life's journey, take the wisdom of these basketball tales to heart. Hold onto your dreams with the courage and strength of a champion, face challenges with the spirit of a hero, make sure to sprinkle some magic along your path and most importantly, have lots of fun along the way! May each step on your path help you to learn about yourself and find even more courage to reach for the stars. I wonder what wonderful story yours will be? Whatever it is, be a star on and off the court, and be yourself all the way through!

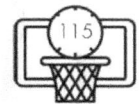

REFERENCES

A dunk and an exclamation that still reverberate. (2013, January 25). *The New York Times.* https://www.nytimes.com/2013/01/25/sports/ncaabasketball/call-by-espn-broadcaster-bill-raftery-on-dunk-by-jerome-lane-still-reverberates.html

Ainbinder, R. (n.d.). *The mysterious story of Michael Jordan's jersey heist.* Sports Tech Biz. https://www.sportstechbiz.com/p/the-mysterious-story-of-michael-jordans

Burton, R. (n.d.-a). *How Vince Carter killed the NBA slam dunk contest.* Bleacher Report. Retrieved July 29, 2023, from https://bleacherreport.com/articles/1081007-how-vince-carter-killed-the-nba-slam-dunk-contest

Burton, R. (n.d.-b). *Ranking the 25 greatest dunks in NBA slam dunk contest history.* Bleacher Report. Retrieved July 29, 2023, from https://bleacherreport.com/articles/1525664-ranking-the-25-greatest-dunks-in-nba-slam-dunk-contest-history

Cambage dunks in Australia's win over Russia. (2012, August 3). ESPN.com. https://www.espn.com/olympics/summer/2012/basketball/story/_/id/8229042/2012-london-olympics-liz-cambage-dunks-australia-win-russia

Dator, J. (2018, January 29). *This Pelicans fan was caught pretending to be a player during warmups.* SBNation.com. https://www.sbnation.com/lookit/2018/1/29/16945454/pelicans-fan-pretends-to-be-player-warmups-video

Dodson, A. (2017, June 1). *On this day in NBA Finals history: "The Mailman doesn't deliver on Sunday."* Andscape. https://andscape.com/features/nba-history-scottie-pippen-karl-malone-1997-finals/

Duffy, T. (n.d.). *The greatest streetballers in NBA history.* Bleacher Report. https://bleacherreport.com/articles/1639789-the-greatest-streetballers-in-nba-history

Gaydos, R. (2022, December 7). *NBA mascot tears down rim on trampoline dunk.* Fox News. https://www.foxnews.com/sports/nba-mascot-tears-down-rim-trampoline-dunk

Gupta, S. (2023, July 31). *Watch: Charles Barkley and Nuggets' mascot Rocky's beef for 30 years compiled in one funny video.* Sportskeeda. https://www.sportskeeda.com/basketball/news-watch-charles-barkley-nuggets-mascot-rocky-s-beef-30-years-compiled-one-funny-video

History.com Editors (2021, October 19). *Villanova wins NCAA basketball title in stunning upset.* HISTORY. https://www.history.com/this-day-in-history/greatest-college-basketball-upsets-villanova-georgetown

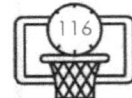

Hoops and laughter: The Harlem Globetrotters. (2018, June 7). American Experience. https://www.pbs.org/wgbh/americanexperience/features/hoops-and-laughter-harlem-globetrotters/

Ke, B. (2020, July 23). *One-Legged basketball player in China goes viral for his incredible three-point shots.* NextShark. https://nextshark.com/luo-xiangjian-one-legged-basketball-player-china

Layden, T. (1985, April 1). *The perfect game.* Sports Illustrated Longform. https://www.si.com/longform/2015/1985/villanova/index.html

Maese, R. (2012, February 16). *Jeremy Lin causes Linsanity in the NBA.* Washington Post. https://www.washingtonpost.com/sports/wizards/jeremy-lin-causes-linsanity-in-the-nba/2012/02/16/gIQAHXugIR_story.html

Merlino, D. (2011, April 29). *Bill Russell: Civil rights hero and inventor of airborne basketball.* Bleacher Report. https://bleacherreport.com/articles/682589-bill-russell-civil-rights-hero-and-inventor-of-airborne-basketball

NBA.com Staff. (2021, September 14). *Top NBA Finals moments: Magic Johnson steps in at center in 1980.* NBA.com. https://www.nba.com/news/history-finals-moments-magic-johnson-steps-in-at-center-in-1980

NBA success stories (II): Allen Iverson. (2021, March 26). Becomeapro. https://www.becomeapro.online/nba-success-stories-ii-allen-iverson-n-93-en

Pat Riley: Biography & facts. (n.d.). Britannica. https://www.britannica.com/biography/Pat-Riley

Quinn, J. (2023, February 14). *On this day: Larry Bird's left-handed game; Edney, Babb born.* Celtics Wire. https://celticswire.usatoday.com/lists/nba-boston-celtics-bird-left-handed-game-edney-babb-born-history-2023/

Rhoden, W. C. (2001, June 4). *Sports of the times: A favorite that became an Underdog.* https://www.nytimes.com/2001/06/04/sports/sports-of-the-times-a-favorite-that-became-an-underdog.html

Sibor, D. (n.d.). *The most inspirational moments and performances in NBA history.* Complex. https://www.complex.com/sports/a/doug-sibor/the-most-inspirational-moments-and-performances-in-nba-history

Sportseasons. (2018, September 24). *The inspiring true story of Jason McElwain.* Sport-Seasons-Blog. https://sport-seasons-blog.com/the-inspiring-story-of-jason/

Superfan: The Nav Bhatia story. (2019). CBC. https://www.cbc.ca/documentaries/specials/superfan-the-nav-bhatia-story-1.6235377

The Naismith Memorial basketball hall of fame: Pat Riley. (n.d.). Hoophall. https://www.hoophall.com/hall-of-famers/pat-riley/

Zweig, M. (n.d.). *A tribute to Pat Riley and his lasting impact in the NBA.* Bleacher Report. https://bleacherreport.com/articles/1650268-a-tribute-to-pat-riley-and-his-lasting-impact-in-the-nba

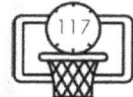

www.ingramcontent.com/pod-product-compliance
Lightning Source LLC
Chambersburg PA
CBHW052157110526
44591CB00012B/1982